Pilates and Parkinson's

Pilates and Parkinson's

Sarah Sessa and Karen Pearce

AEON

First published in 2016 by Muswell Hill Press.

This new edition published in 2019 by
Aeon Books Ltd

British Library Cataloguing in Publication Data

A C.I.P. for this book is available from the British Library

ISBN-13: 978-1-91327-412-2

www.aeonbooks.co.uk

Contents

PART TWO

Foreword

By Alan Herdman

Sarah Sessa and Karen Pearce have produced a book *Pilates and Parkinson's* that should be in every Pilates's instructors bag or on their bedside table. Parkinson's is introduced in a way that is clear and concise. The reader is guided through Parkinson's allowing them to understand all the aspects of the condition. The explanation of how Parkinson's affects movement and function is particularly important to Pilates instructors. Every Pilates instructor will know the background and principles of the Pilate's technique. I would recommend that they read this section and re-visit these principles, which will help them to understand the exercises that are not strictly the Pilates exercises that they know from their training.

The exercise routines in part two are excellent. Although a programme using the mat and apparatus is recommended, the instructor who is only mat trained will find the mat exercises extremely beneficial to clients with Parkinson's. Having used these exercises in my studios for many years I can guarantee that they work. I have read this excellent book as a Pilates teacher and educator and I know that it is an important addition to the teachers library. It is equally important as a companion to the client with Parkinson's as background information about their condition and as a useful homework book.

Introduction

Although I am far from happy with the diagnosis, I now feel I am doing something to help myself Ray, 2011.

The Purpose of This Book

We decided to write this book to provide a useful guide to two groups of people. Firstly, for those diagnosed with Parkinson's who are looking for a safe form of exercise that could work for them. There are lots of Pilates books out there, but none specifically related to Parkinson's that provide exercises specific and appropriate to this condition. Over the past few years we have seen a number of clients coming through our studio doors with Parkinson's who have felt the enormous benefits of Pilates. They tell us how their increased flexibility and strength as well as their improved balance and walking have helped them to remain independent. Secondly, we hope this book will also be enjoyed by Pilates instructors who are wondering how they can best help a client who comes in with a diagnosis of Parkinson's.

There are few, if any scientific trials that investigate the use of Pilates in the management of Parkinson's. We have therefore used information that we sourced when writing up a recent case study, together with our physiotherapy knowledge and the experiences that we have had with our clients in our day-to-day clinical practice to inform the basis of the exercises and advice in this book.

Being diagnosed with a progressive condition is difficult to say the least; a person may feel shock and sadness, a loss of control, or that their life is entirely in the hands of the doctors and medication. Many people enter a period of denial, and may require support to help come to terms with the diagnosis. One client said:

I am told by friends that I became very detached and quiet for three months after being diagnosed. Prior to my diagnosis I had arranged to do the GR20, a twelve day hike along the length of the mountains of

Corsica. It was doing this that helped me out of my depression and made me realise that there was life after Parkinson's.

Finding an exercise regime that could work by reducing symptoms such as weakness, poor movement, muscle rigidity, stiffness and poor balance, can allow you to feel more in control. It is something YOU can do to help manage the condition. We believe this approach not only provides physical benefits, but also a greater sense of wellbeing and relaxation.

In this book we offer the reader an overview of physiotherapy, exercise and Pilates in relation to Parkinson's followed by clear exercise programmes that can either be made part of your daily routine or compliment your Pilates class if you already attend one. There is a chapter describing exercises using small equipment and another chapter on the Pilates machines for those attending a studio with such apparatus. The programmes described are not exhaustive, as there are a large number of exercises in the Pilates repertoire that might be suitable for you. We explain the reasons why certain specific movements and exercises are especially good for Parkinson's to help you to understand better, and choose from these and other resources.

Once you start Pilates you will quickly catch the Pilates bug and miss it when you don't do it. You will find yourself carrying out these exercises whilst waiting for a bus or making a cup of tea, and it will become a way of life for you. To begin with you might find Pilates very gentle, but you will be surprised how a seemingly innocent looking exercise is actually quite a challenge. If you are consistent with exercising, before you know it your core will be stronger and your flexibility so improved that you might become more flexible than you have ever been before. Furthermore, because there is always another Pilates exercise to learn you will never be bored!

More than anything we hope this book will be a useful tool to help you along your journey towards a fitter, healthier lifestyle; a guide to let you know you *can* do something to help manage the physical symptoms of the Parkinson's.

Balance of Body: The Pilates Method –
A Balance of Body and Mind

Joseph Pilates was born in 1883 in Germany: he was a sickly child and grew up determined to improve his physical ability. He came to England just before the First World War as a circus performer. When war broke out, because of his nationality he was interned at a hospital where he was required to offer rehabilitation to war veterans. His famous Universal Reformer machine was originally invented by attaching springs to hospital beds to allow those confined to bed to exercise. After the war, Pilates returned to Germany, and soon after that moved to New York where he devised an exercise regime called Contrology.[1] He developed this regime from watching animals stretch, from practicing self-defence, acrobatics, boxing, and eventually from working with some of the leading ballet dancers of the time. Contrology was based on the principles of muscle balance, core strength and agility – an exercise system that required thought too. Joseph Pilates felt strongly that his exercise was to be used in everyday life – as a way of life!

The Pilates that is practiced today has the advantage of being used and improved by physiotherapists and other health and exercise professionals; as we gain greater knowledge of the human body these techniques are improved. We talk about the Principles of Pilates but it must be noted that they were not directly developed by Pilates himself but by instructors and the Pilates community. For this reason they may differ slightly depending on your source of information. However the concept and message remain the same – *A Balance of Body and Mind.*

The Six Principles

Breath

A good breathing pattern will stop your breath becoming tense and shallow, which can cause even simple things such as climbing stairs to feel difficult. Learning to control your breathing will allow movements to become more natural and relaxed.

With Pilates exercises we mainly use a lateral breathing technique, which is a breath into the sides of the ribcage as opposed to expanding the abdomen (or pushing out the tummy). This mirrors our natural way of breathing and enables the deep abdominal muscles to be engaged on both inhalation and exhalation, which helps to stabilise the pelvic girdle and strengthen the core muscles

Concentration

Having to isolate certain muscles also focuses the mind. Thinking about the breathing pattern, the muscles being activated and the correct alignment of the body will improve concentration. As you become more proficient at the exercises you will begin to realise how the mind can control our movements – it's just a matter of connecting mind to body.

Centre

Strength comes from a central point of your body, which is often called your *core*. To feel that your body is centred means that the muscles are balanced and the core muscles are strong. This allows you to maintain a correct posture and undertake everyday activities without causing injury to vulnerable places such as the spine. For people with Parkinson's, this would particularly help your lower back area, which is prone to stiffness, weakness and then pain.

Practicing Pilates will improve the way that you stand and eliminate the muscular pain caused by bad posture. As your central core muscles become stronger, the exercises should also help preserve your balance responses.

Control

When practicing the Pilates exercises regularly you will gradually improve to achieve the desired amount of control. The muscles should work in better harmony so that the stronger ones don't dominate, and you will start to feel in control of your movements. For many people, the programme of exercises will feel more natural and require less of a conscious effort over time. For some people with Parkinson's however, you may need to be taught ways to remember to control your movement.

Precision

Pilates exercises consist mainly of small and very subtle movements; precision is more important than repetition. We can get into bad postural habits and allow some muscles to become over strong and tight, and others weak and underused.

Acquiring an understanding of which muscles should be working and isolating these muscles will correct these issues. Although it may seems difficult at first, the ability to isolate muscles improves with practise and once mastered can be taken into every aspect of daily life.

Flow

As we get older our joints start to stiffen, we have a tendency to move less and so we lose some flexibility. If we keep our joints moving and our muscles stretched, however, we can continue to stay flexible, maintain an upright posture and retain agility into old age. This is all the more achievable if a Pilates routine is practised regularly and becomes a way of life.

PART ONE

CHAPTER 1

Some Core Concepts

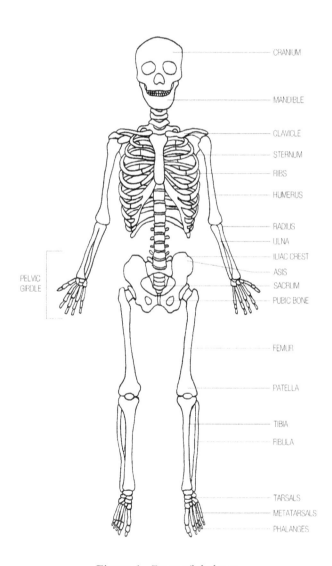

Figure 1. Front of skeleton.

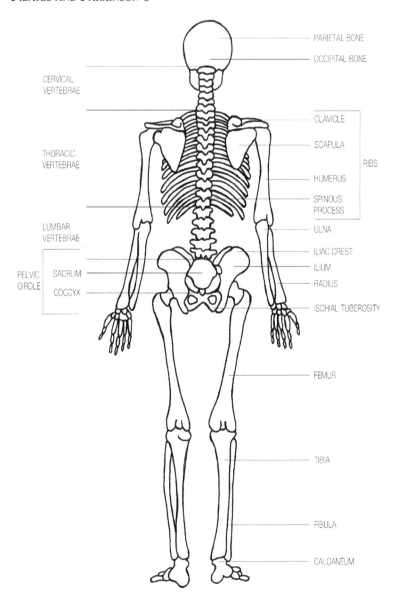

Figure 2. Back of skeleton.

The Vertebral Column or Spine

The vertebral column is made up of 33 small, but strong bones (the vertebrae) joined together by interconnecting joints and reinforced by ligaments and muscles. The vertebrae are divided into groups: the 7 cervical vertebrae of the neck, 12 thoracic vertebrae of your mid back to which your ribcage is attached, 5 lumbar vertebrae of your lower back, 5 fused sacral vertebra (the sacrum) and 3–4 coccygeal vertebrae (coccyx or tailbone). The design of the individual vertebrae differs depending on where they are within the spine and what is required of them.

The vertebral column has several functions including the housing of the spinal cord in a natural canal or space down the middle. This protects the spinal cord, a vital structure, which contains nerve tracts that run from the brain to the rest of the body carrying important information back and forth. The vertebral column provides attachment for many muscles and ligaments, and the bony structure supports the rest of the skeleton – especially the weight of the upper body. This function allows us to move in different directions: bending forwards (flexion), bending backwards (extension), side bending, and rotation (twisting). The motion between each section or between two vertebrae may not be much but the sum of all these small movements up and down the column produces a significant amount of movement.

Neutral Pelvis

In this book and many other Pilates books we talk about a *neutral pelvis*. Your pelvic girdle connects the vertebral column (your backbone or spine) to your legs. The two (left and right) sides of the pelvis are joined together at the front by the pubic symphysis (pubic joint) and at the back by the sacro iliac joints. Each side of the pelvis is made up of the ilium, ischium and pubic bones.

The pelvis is a very strong, rigid ring of bone that has to transmit a lot of weight whilst allowing the different parts of the body to be held correctly. This function prevents weakness or injury during movements such as lifting, walking, standing up or getting in and out of bed. The pelvis provides attachment for many powerful and supportive muscles and ligaments, protects our pelvic organs and forms the birth canal in females. We expect a lot from the pelvis: not only does it have to be strong and rigid but it also has to move subtly during many activities. If the muscles that are attached to it aren't working correctly then the pelvis will no longer be aligned properly, putting stress on other joints such as the lower back, hips, knees and feet. As some muscles weaken, others will tighten creating an imbalance in its optimal working position.

The neutral pelvis position is when the pelvis is held in such a way that all the muscles attached to it are working in harmony so that joints are supported and there is no excessive strain in other places.

So how do we find neutral pelvis?

There are many different ways to do this, but a good place to start would be in the Pilates rest position, with you lying on the floor, on your back with your hips and knees bent. Your feet should be on the floor, hip width apart.

Think about your lower back and the contact it has with the floor or mat. Is there a big curve in the small of your back, or is your lower back flattened down so there is no gap at all?

Neither of these positions are what you want; you are aiming to feel a gentle curve in the small of your back that will almost allow a flat hand to fit under it.

Next, put your fingers on the bony points you can feel at the front of your hips. These points are known as the anterior superior iliac spines (ASIS), and provide attachment for muscles. Although they are really part of the pelvis, for the purpose of this book we will refer to them as your hip bones. Keep one hand on a hip bone and place the other hand on your pubic joint where the 2 pubic bones meet. The 2 hip bones and the pubic joint should be in the same horizontal or flat plane, so the pubic bone should not be higher or lower than the hip bones or vice versa. When you are standing, these 3 bony points should once again be in the same plane (this time the vertical plane). This is neutral pelvis (also neutral spine).

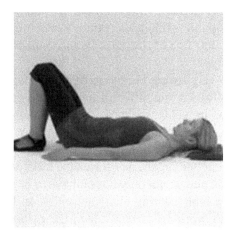

Figure 3. The Pilates rest position.

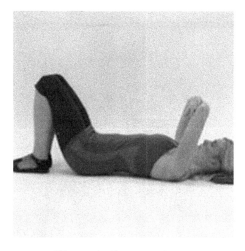

Figure 4. Curve too large.

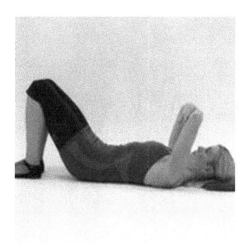

Figure 5. Back too flattened.

Core Muscles

Anyone that does Pilates quickly becomes attuned to their bodies and can't help but register those muscles that the instructor keeps mentioning. You are taught to feel where they are and whether you are engaging them correctly and at the right time. You therefore become aware of tightness, whether (and which) muscles are overactive as this will prevent other muscles from moving properly. You will learn about the importance of muscle balance and how the muscles need to work together to maintain a well aligned, pain free posture and free fluid movements that are more efficient.

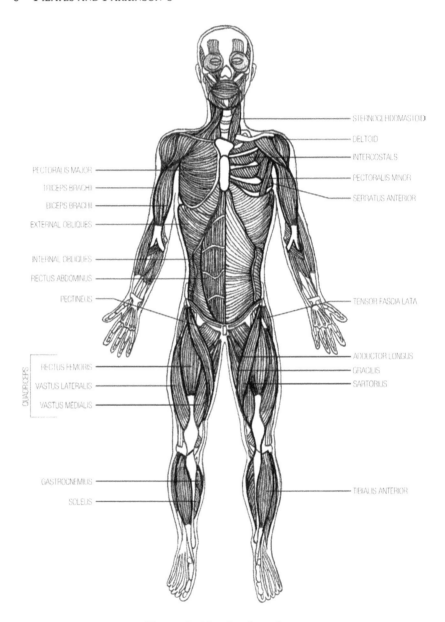

Figure 6. Muscles from front.

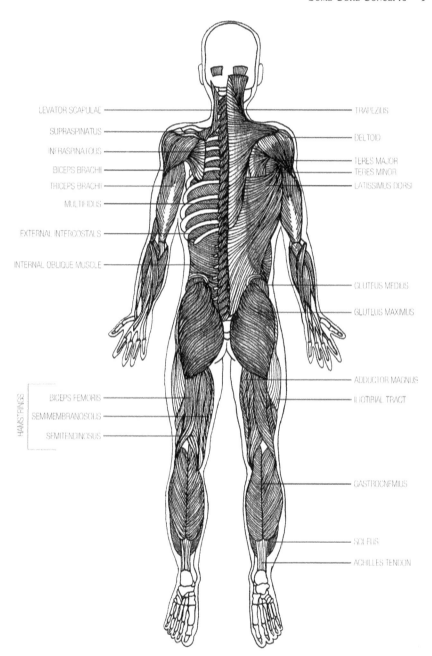

LEVATOR SCAPULAE

SUPRASPINATUS

INFRASPINATOUS

BICEPS BRACHII

TRICEPS BRACHII

MULTIFIDUS

EXTERNAL INTERCOSTALS

INTERNAL OBLIQUE MUSCLE

TRAPEZIUS

DELTOID

TERES MAJOR
TERES MINOR

LATISSIMUS DORSI

GLUTEUS MEDIUS

GLUTEUS MAXIMUS

ADDUCTOR MAGNUS

ILIOTIBIAL TRACT

HAMSTRINGS

BICEPS FEMORIS

SEMIMEMBRANOSOUS

SEMITENDINOSUS

GASTROCNEMIUS

SOLEUS

ACHILLES TENDON

Figure 7. Muscles from back.

Muscles that are close to the surface such as your rectus abdominus and erector spinae are powerful movers whereas those that are close to the joints and bones – *the core muscles* – are more stabilising.

Pilates is holistic and we aim to achieve muscle balance throughout the body but there is a major emphasis on having a strong core or centre. By this we mean those muscles that protect and stabilise the back; these muscles are found around the abdomen, the lower back and the pelvis. During Pilates exercises we engage our core muscles allowing stability around our centre so that we can move our arms and legs freely and efficiently.

The main muscle that we consciously engage when thinking of the core is the transversus abdominus (TA). This is not to say that it is the only important stabilising muscle but they are a good starting point. The transversus abdominus is the deepest of the lateral abdominal muscles and wraps around our lower waist like a firm, supportive corset. As it comes round to the front it inserts into the central linea alba, a strong tendinous strip where all the abdominal muscles meet. The fibres of this muscle run across your stomach area like a wide elastic belt, providing support and gentle compression to the abdominal organs and support to your lower back. As the TA engages so too does another muscle at the back called multifidus, which is also an important core muscle and found close to the vertebrae underneath erector spinae.

> *"Breathe in to prepare, breathe out, lift up with the pelvic floor, draw in the lateral abdominals………."* – Our mantra!!

As you draw in the lateral abdominals the TA becomes engaged. It shouldn't be a big suck in of the abdominal muscles; feel the connection of the bottom of the rib cage towards your pubic bone and imagine you are drawing the 2 hip bones together towards the centre. Remember these muscles only need to work with low-level stamina to provide stability, so do not strain yourself to achieve the position. They do not need to activate strongly to produce large forceful movements such as is needed from the quadriceps to straighten the knee or the biceps to bend the elbow. This low-level contraction needs to be about 30% of the maximum contraction that you can do. If you suck in your lower tummy hard, this is 100% and you won't be able to maintain it, you only need a 1/3 of this, perhaps feeling hardly like a contraction at all.

The pelvic floor muscles are also part of the core and stretch from the pubic bone to the tailbone. We usually think of them as a sling from the front passage to the back passage that also stretches crossways between the two sitting bones or ischial tuberosities. The pelvic floor muscles provide support for our pelvic organs and are also very important for continence of both faeces and urine and also for sexual function. Together with

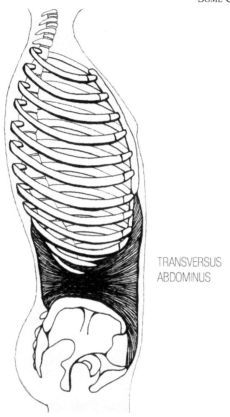

TRANSVERSUS
ABDOMINUS

Figure 8. Transversus abdominus.

the abdominals and back muscles they help to stabilise the spine. Both men and women have pelvic floor muscles.

> "*Breathe in to prepare, breathe out, pull up the pelvic floor and draw in the lateral abdominals………*"

With these three core muscles engaged (TA, pelvic floor, multifidus) and your pelvis and lower back in correct alignment you have a better chance of performing Pilates exercises correctly and having improved posture, strength and flexibility.

If it sounds complicated, don't worry. As you do the exercises in our programmes this gentle engagement of the core muscles becomes easier.

Muscle Balance

Pilates isn't just about the core. We aim to condition all the muscles throughout our body, trying to get them to function and work together correctly. Muscles have different types of fibres depending on their function and what is needed of them. They are described as three types of muscles.

Local Stabilisers

These muscles lie deep to the joint providing stability and support. They are designed for endurance and produce a gentle, low-level contraction that can be sustained. Think of these muscles as *whispering*; they need to keep whispering all the time without getting tired. There are many examples of local stabilisers but some that we often mention in the Pilates studio are transversus abdominus, internal obliques (underneath external obliques), multifidus, gluteus medius, lower fibres of trapezius and deep neck flexors. These muscles are responsible for maintaining correct posture but sometimes they do not work as they should, perhaps due to pain or increased loading, maybe because of a degenerative process, as in arthritis, or a condition like Parkinson's, where the muscle tone is affected. As a result they no longer provide the stability to the joints that they ought to.

Global (or Secondary) Stabilisers

These muscles are not as deep as the local stabilising muscles and their function is to help to control movement. They turn on and off depending on the movement that is taking place rather than providing a sustained contraction. If we stick with the analogy of the local stability muscles fibres whispering, then, the muscle fibres of the global stabilisers should be *talking*. They are powerful and can absorb a large amount of force. Examples are gluteus maximus, external obliques, the quadriceps and some upper fibres of trapezius. If these fibres don't produce enough force then they will exhibit lack of control and become shaky.

Global Mobilisers

These muscles work under high load and are *SHOUTING*!!! They are built to produce power but lack endurance. They are superficial and can build up tension quickly. Examples of these powerful mobilisers are the hamstrings, rectus abdominus, erector spinae and the fibres of upper trapezius. These muscles can easily become tight perhaps due to overuse or disease such as Parkinson's or stroke that affects muscle tone.

Several muscles can have two roles, as we see with the upper fibres of trapezius; they can work as a global stabiliser or mobiliser depending on the situation.

Good Postural Alignment

Posture is the position that we hold our body in when up against gravity. We think of posture in sitting, standing or lying. *Good posture* is the position where there is as little strain as possible on the muscles, ligaments, bones and joints. We want the bones and joints to be correctly aligned in order to avoid pain and injury. Sometimes differences in posture can be structural where the bones are incorrectly aligned from birth: for example if someone is born with a curve (scoliosis) of their spine. Or it can be functional such as a posture adapted to an occupation or activity: perhaps sitting for a long time at a computer, carrying a baby on one hip or lots of driving. The degenerative process of Parkinson's can affect posture so that changes to the muscles can to lead to altered pull on bones and joints. Each person varies in the way that they hold themselves but very broadly speaking there are four main categories: lordotic, flat back, kyphotic and sway back. Some people may have elements of more than one posture type. From the following pictures, can you relate to any particular type? Bare this in mind as you read through this book and see if you can gently correct any elements of poor posture that you might have noted about yourself.

Factors Influencing Posture:

- Your genetic make-up.
- Habitual positions, occupation, repetitive movements, particular activities.
- A condition such as Parkinson's, stroke, osteoporosis, arthritis.
- Trauma.
- Altered muscle activity or muscle imbalance that can be due to any of the above.

With a condition such as Parkinson's, which affects the tone of muscle, your posture can become more bent forwards. Muscles therefore tighten which makes movement harder, while some muscles stretch and weaken. The combined consequence of this tightening and weakening is that some people might experience pain. Being aware of good posture and trying to maintain it will really help you. Once you get settled into a routine with your Pilates practice, you will find that you are holding your body in a better position without having to think about it as much, or by using a simple cue to jog your memory.

Your Posture

Stand in front of a full-length mirror and have a look at your posture. If you are alone, do this in your underwear and bare feet, so you can see your

LORDOTIC
POSTURE

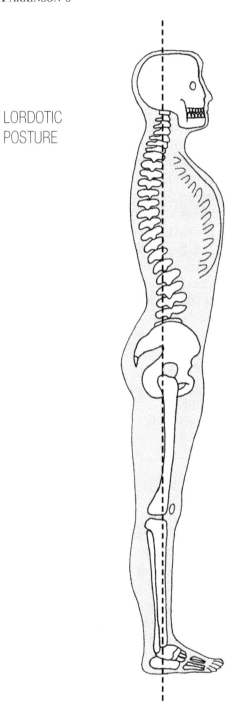

Figure 9. Lordotic.

KYPHOTIC
POSTURE

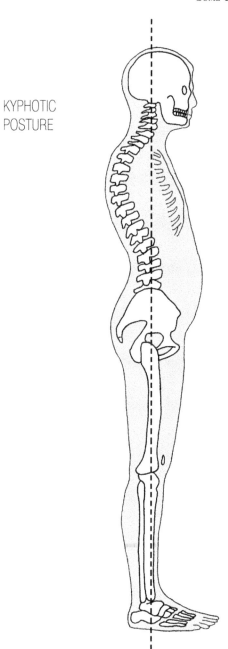

Figure 10. Kyphotic.

FLAT-BACK
POSTURE

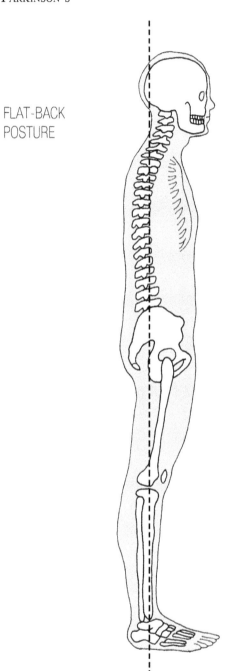

Figure 11. Flat back.

SWAY BACK
POSTURE

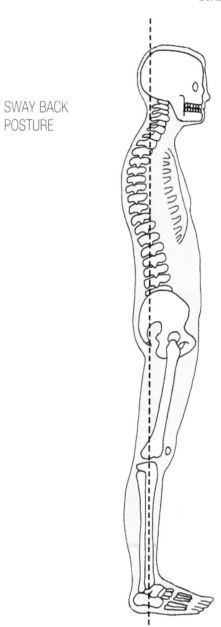

Figure 12. Sway back.

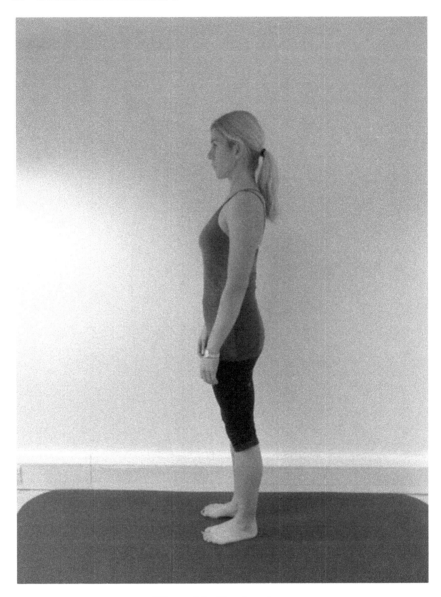

Figure 13. Good posture.

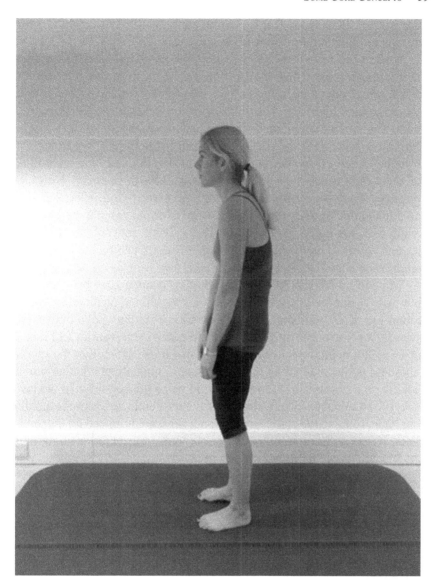

Figure 14. Poor posture.

body clearly. Place your feet hip-width apart, so that they are underneath your knees, which in turn should be underneath your hips.

Start at the feet. They should be almost parallel. Check to see if one leg is turned out more than the other, and if so, try to correct this. Are your feet too rolled out or too rolled in? For example, if you have flat feet or are your arches too high, then you will place more pressure on the shins or the knees. Think of a triangle on the base of each foot: the top of the triangle is right through the heel and the two points at the bottom of the triangle are through the ball of the foot and the base of the little toe. You want to feel that the weight is equally distributed through these three points. Now close your eyes (have something close by to hold onto if your balance is poor) and think about whether the weight is even over the triangle; perhaps your weight feels too far backwards or forwards. Try to concentrate on the contact that your feet have with the floor, and really try to feel that your body weight is equally distributed between both feet.

Moving up the legs first to the knees, try a small knee bend and think about what your knees are doing. The kneecap should be directed over the second toe when you bend. Do they do this or do they poke outwards or inwards? As you come up to the hips and pelvis, you want to feel that the pelvis is in a neutral position as we discussed earlier, so that the two hip bones and pubic bone are in the same plane. Think about whether you are sticking your bottom out too much giving you a greater curve in the lower back, or the opposite. There should be a very gentle curve in the small of your back. If the curve is too large, greater pressure is placed on the lumbar joints. If you do have an increased curve, tuck your tailbone slight under and feel a lengthening in your lower back.

Come up to your stomach and ribs: your deep abdominals and pelvic floor should be engaged a little, your ribs are soft, not flared and sticking out. Gently open up your chest and feel your collar bones widen.

Your arms should hang relaxed beside you, your shoulders shouldn't be hunched up or rounded forwards; if they are, draw them back a little but don't squeeze them back. Some people with Parkinson's who are starting to bend forward, hold their arms back as compensation for weaker upper back muscles. Be aware of this when you do this part of the postural exercise. Concentrate on your shoulders moving backwards, opening your chest, but don't let the top of your arms pull back like a soldier. The back of your neck should be long, and your chin drawn down slightly – think about holding a ripe soft peach under your chin, you want just enough hold to stop it dropping but you don't want to bruise it.

When you feel you are standing nicely, place your hands on the bottom of your rib cage at the front and take a slow, relaxed breath in. Feel that your lower rig cage and abdomen expand a little under your hands but that your upper chest barely moves – no puffing up! Then gently breathe out through your mouth and feel your lower rib cage and abdomen relax in again.

Summary

- Pilates is a holistic exercise regime that is popular and easily accessible and may be of help to you if you have Parkinson's.
- Start by finding neutral pelvis and thinking about your core.
- Muscles differ in the way they are designed depending on the function required of them. Ideally we want harmony and balance between the different groups, and that they are moved in such a way as not to strain them or create tension.
- It is important to know what good postural alignment is and how to achieve it, as this can be affected in Parkinson's.

CHAPTER 2

Parkinson's: A Brief Overview

What is Parkinson's?

Parkinson's is a degenerative neurological disorder, with symptoms that tend to appear gradually and will progress over time. Parkinson's occurs in about 1 in 500 people in the UK with slightly more men than women being affected. Onset is usually after the age of 50 although Parkinson's is sometimes diagnosed in people under the age of 40. We saw this with *Back to the Future* star, Michael J Fox, who was only 30 years old when diagnosed. Most symptoms of Parkinson's are known as *motor symptoms*, which refer to movement problems. However, there may also be non-motor symptoms, including bladder and bowel difficulties, psychological changes, such as changes in mood and emotional response. Parkinson's is sometimes associated with cognitive difficulty, for example with face recognition, remembering names, or retaining new information. There may also be sensory disturbances and the cardiovascular system may be affected.[2] Everyone with Parkinson's has a different experience and set of symptoms, with varying speeds of progression of the condition. The cause of Parkinson's is not clear – in a small number of cases, it is directly linked to a genetic cause. But we do know that there is a decrease in a brain chemical called *dopamine* in all people with Parkinson's. At present there is no cure, BUT many of the movement symptoms and their consequences can be improved through exercise such as Pilates.

The Scientific Part: What is happening in the brain?

Although different changes occur throughout the brains of people who have Parkinson's, which is why people demonstrate such a variety of symptoms, we will concentrate on the role of dopamine. This is a chemical found throughout the body, but it has a particular function in the brain. It acts as a neurotransmitter, a substance released between nerve cells in order to set off electrical signals along our nerves to different areas of our body. Deep within

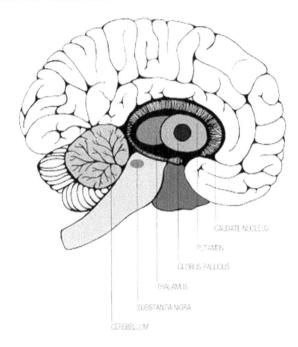

CAUDATE NUCLEUS

PUTAMEN

GLOBUS PALLIDUS

THALAMUS

SUBSTANTIA NIGRA

CEREBELLUM

Figure 15. The Basal ganglia.

the brain is a structure called the *substantia nigra* that produces dopamine, and in Parkinson's it is the cells found in the substantia nigra and its pathways that are destroyed. The substantia nigra produces the dopamine that is needed in a part of the brain called the basal ganglia, a group of nuclei concerned with the production of smooth, well controlled, automatic movement. These nuclei talk to other parts of the brain, gathering information and then sending out the signals required to produce automatic, and fluid movement.

Dopamine isn't just used in the basal ganglia but also in other parts of the brain so when the dopamine levels are disturbed, as in Parkinson's, there may also be difficulty with other aspects of functioning due to the normal balance with other neurotransmitters becoming compromised. Thus many of the non-motor symptoms that we mentioned previously might be affected in this indirect way – they do not depend primarily on dopamine but the balance of the neurotransmitters is altered and this subtly affects function.

Onset, Diagnosis and Stages of Parkinson's

For each person the way in which symptoms appear will differ. Onset may be slow and gradual, especially in those diagnosed at a younger age, perhaps initially with just a feeling of stiffness in a limb, or a slight tremor of one hand. Some people may have Parkinson's for up to a couple of years before a diagnosis is confirmed by a specialist neurologist to whom you will have been referred by your GP. The neurologist performs a clinical examination looking for specific signs of Parkinson's such as tremor, slow movement (bradykinesia) or muscle rigidity. It is important that the diagnosis is correct so that the appropriate treatment can be started. If the neurologist is unsure and needs added tests to confirm the diagnosis, you may be sent for a scan that looks at the structures of the brain, such as a DaTSCAN (dopamine transporter scan), which can detect loss of the dopamine producing cells.

Medical Treatment

Although this book is concerned principally with exercise and Pilates as one way to manage Parkinson's, it is important to consider its role alongside other aspects of medical care in the management of Parkinson's. [3] Despite the lack of a cure for Parkinson's there is plenty of research going on trying to better understand the causes, and treatments of the condition. Medications may be used to increase the levels of dopamine in the brain depending on your symptoms and stage of Parkinson's. One of the most common types of Parkinson's drug is Levodopa (brand names are Madopar or Sinemet), which the brain converts into dopamine. As there are many combinations of Parkinson's medicines, your doctor and specialist Parkinson's nurse should monitor these and make alterations depending on your symptoms.

There are also surgical options too such as a technique called Deep Brain Stimulation (DBS), where electrodes are placed inside your brain and produce an electric current which can change some of the signals that cause the symptoms of Parkinson's.

Make sure you are involved with decisions about your treatments, as they can have a wide impact on the way you live. Discuss your thoughts and experiences with your doctor and nurse. For example, one client reported that if he went out to a social event in the evening and had taken his normal dose of medication, his movement became more erratic (dyskinesic) due to the change in routine, but this was much improved if he only took half the dose.

Everyone is different and one drug regime might not be suitable or everyone, your doctor and nurse can help you manage your medication so that it is right for you. We would advise you look up information regarding investigations, such as scans, and any treatments on the Parkinson's UK website. They also have a lot of information about the management of the non-motor symptoms, many of which do not respond to dopamine-based interventions.

Summary

- Parkinson's is a degenerative neurological condition that results in movement problems, especially of automatic movements, as well as a variety of non-motor symptoms.
- Lack of a neurotransmitter in the brain called dopamine is the main cause of the movement disorder.
- There is no cure for Parkinson's at present. Medical treatment consists of drugs to increase dopamine in the brain, or other medications to help manage non-motor symptoms such as bladder and bowel problems, blood pressure and mood or cognitive-related symptoms. Surgery such as Deep Brain Stimulation can be offered in some cases.

CHAPTER 3

Parkinson's and Physiotherapy

How does Parkinson's affect Movement and Function?

Combine the motor and non-motor symptoms together and we have a recipe for a more sedentary life, which in turn may worsen existing symptoms, or cause complications such as constipation, falls, poor balance, higher risk of osteoporosis (bone thinning) and problems with one's cardiovascular and metabolic systems. The prevalence of osteoporosis in Parkinson's is higher, perhaps because of decreased activity and muscle strength, low body weight and also vitamin D deficiency.[4]

Motor Symptoms

Slowness of movement (bradykinesia), rigidity of muscles, tremor and balance problems are the principle symptoms of Parkinson's. As muscles become stiffer and your movement slower, you may feel yourself a little bent over with a more kyphotic posture. You are no longer standing up as straight, which in turn makes some muscles even tighter and others weaker because they are not being used in the normal way. The trunk becomes less mobile because of the rigidity, and the brain may not process sensory information as well as it did. All these factors combine to result in slower movements in general and a marked difficulty in correcting your position when needing to maintain balance. Furthermore, the 'fine motor activities' such as writing and fastening buttons can become more difficult, as well as actions such as reaching and keeping hold of objects. Movements that require you to rotate (twist), such as getting in and out of bed, or that need speed and power, such as getting up off a chair or low sofa, can also become more challenging as muscles and joints stiffen.

The basal ganglia are also responsible for automatic control. When they are not working properly, secondary to the lack of dopamine, movements that do not ordinarily require thinking about, such as walking, become more difficult. Sometimes just being more *mindful* of a movement (mindfulness forms a large part of Pilates) and really thinking about the action before doing it can help.

Functional Activities

Parkinson's and the resultant slowed processing within the basal ganglia can cause decreased mobility of the trunk and some impairment of balance mechanisms – which in turn can increase your risk of falling.

Let's use walking as an example to consider the impact of these things. Think about the way you walk, or watch a friend or your partner walking, and you will see that it isn't just our legs that move. Our bodies rotate a little for counterbalance and our arms swing gently when we walk, helping us to be as efficient and as balanced as possible. For people with Parkinson's, we know that each step length shortens due to a combination of bradykinesia and rigidity, so you may not stride out as you once used to. The rigidity in the trunk means that you do not move as freely as you did, so your walking speed becomes slower and walking becomes more effortful. Regarding your own experience, are you aware that you are shuffling when you are walking? Are you freezing (a feeling of being glued to the spot), or do you come to a stop at a doorway or obstacle? You may find it hard to get going and once you do, you find you cannot stop. Doing two things at once (dual tasking) can also become difficult, so although you might feel you are perfectly fine walking down the high street, when your phone rings you might notice that you struggle to hold a conversation at the same time as walking.

Exercise, Physiotherapy and Parkinson's

Physiotherapists have always worked closely with people with Parkinson's, providing exercise programmes and balance re-education as well as working on their walking and general function.

As physiotherapists we strive to provide our patients or clients with the best treatment that we believe is effective. Treatments, as far as possible, are based on sound evidence, hopefully proven through research, but sometimes through the individual's experience and our own. In other words, physios endeavour to provide clients with the best management and advice available and also bear this in mind when sharing knowledge with colleagues such as Pilates Instructors. It is very satisfying to be able to give a Pilates exercise programme to studio clients that sticks to the all-important physiotherapy principles. The exercise programmes devised for this book are all based on the principles for physiotherapy set out by the Dutch/European Physiotherapy Guidelines (KNGF), which physiotherapists throughout the UK and mainland Europe are encouraged to follow.[5] These Guidelines are based on a systematic review of the research evidence and supplemented with clinical expertise as well as the views of people with Parkinson's. They support optimal care for those with Parkinson hence, for this book we have thought of exercises that adhere to these guidelines.

Being told you have Parkinson's can be incredibly hard emotionally, and it can take time to come to terms with the diagnosis. But at the point of diagnosis, at this early stage, there is a window of opportunity to improve your physical capabilities. You will need to make sure you remain as active as possible, aiming for a good level of exercise, possibly even improving your exercise capacity if you are not that physically active. This is the time to get in as best shape as you can. Think about what activities you enjoy; whether it is walking, gardening, cycling or dancing. Make time each week for your chosen activity. Guidelines specifically for people with Parkinson's, as well as the department of health guidance, suggest regular (preferably 3–5 times weekly) exercise for 4 weeks can reduce functional limitation, and after 8 weeks physical capacity is improved. There are different management strategies for the different stages of Parkinson's but in this book we want to consider in particular the first stage of the condition, in which there is the greatest window of opportunity. At this point in order to maintain the best physical conditions possible physiotherapists will be aiming to *prevent inactivity*. We want to give our clients confidence to move correctly, and to work on balance in order to reduce worries about falling. The aim is to prevent for as long as possible, or to improve as much as possible, poor muscle strength and any reduced joint range.

How do we do this? Improve, Preserve, Prevent

Improve reaching, grasping and manipulating moving objects.
Improve balance.
Improve gait.
Preserve or improve physical function.
Preserve independence.
Prevent falls.

Physiotherapists will thoroughly assess a client's physical ability and design a treatment plan specific to each individual. Depending on your symptoms they will give you exercise programmes, practice activities and use hands-on manual therapy to help with stiff joints and muscles, which in turn will aid freer movement. Through these treatments they are aiming to help you stay as independent as possible with functional movements so you can best live the life that you want to lead.

There are numerous ways in which we might combine physiotherapy, exercise and a Pilates programme. We might target walking problems, getting in and out of bed, on and off chairs or low sofas as well reaching activities and fine motor tasks, such doing up buttons. Providing cues and avoiding dual tasking can sometimes help with arm and hand activities. We will help you work on your posture and how to become more conscious of how to correct any imbalances. By providing verbal and visual feedback, for example using a mirror, you will be able to see what is going on more easily. Balance re-education or maintenance will involve wobble boards, football, basket-ball or inventing challenging walking tasks. We may give our clients external cues if they are finding it hard to initiate movement automatically. An example would be giving verbal cues or description; most of our clients have the sound of their physio's voice as a permanent fixture in their mind! We might use a metronome to pace your walking or we may position masking tape on the floor to aid stepping. These cues can improve performance of activities and function. Part of being a physiotherapist is being inventive. We will encourage the patient to be more mindful of what they are doing, so they may take a more cognitive approach if they are finding automatic movements difficult.

In reality, after the initial diagnosis with Parkinson's, few people are assessed by a physiotherapist and offered a weekly exercise programme. But if you have a specific problem such as difficulty with walking or falls, or perhaps joints that are stiff and painful, then it might be worth you talking to your GP or Parkinson's Nurse Specialist to enquire whether a referral to a physiotherapist is necessary. Finding a Pilates class or studio that you can attend for weekly sessions may be easier to achieve, as can learning a home exercise programme that you can fit into your daily routine to practice regularly.

Summary

- Motor and non-motor symptoms of Parkinson's will eventually lead to poor mobility function and secondary complications.
- You may experience particular problems with transfers, mobility, balance and fine motor activities.
- Movements that are under automatic control are the most likely to become harder.
- You may experience 'freezing' and difficulty with dual tasking, especially where tasks require that you think and move at the same time.
- Physiotherapists can work with people with Parkinson's, particularly to improve mobility, flexibility and balance, as well as offering exercise programmes to maintain or improve aspects of fitness.

- Your GP or Parkinson's Nurse Specialist may not automatically refer you to a physiotherapist for a maintenance exercise programme, so please discuss the possibility with them.
- Physiotherapists across Europe work and communicate together to produce evidence about the optimum management of Parkinson's clients. Exercise is a really important part of this management.
- A Pilates programme run by instructors that have experience with Parkinson's clients and who know which exercises work and why, will be extremely beneficial.

CHAPTER 4

Pilates for Parkinson's

Why Pilates is Good for Parkinson's

We have discussed the Pilates Method and its recognised benefits in earlier chapters, so now it is time to talk about how these principles can be applied when someone has Parkinson's.

Pilates is a holistic exercise technique concentrating on strength (particularly the core), flexibility, balance, co-ordination, correct breathing and stress relief, all of which are really important when it comes to managing Parkinson's. The huge repertoire of exercises means you will never be bored as there are several ways of doing an exercise to achieve the same benefits. Physiotherapists that also specialise in Pilates use the technique within rehabilitation populations to retrain strength from the core outwards in order to achieve better alignment and prevent recurrence of neurological, musculoskeletal and postural conditions.[6] With neurological conditions we use Pilates to help improve co-ordination, proprioception (the sense of where your joints/limbs are in space), lengthen tight muscles and improve balance. Exercise regimes that work on balance, strength and flexibility such as Pilates and Tai Chi can really help in the prevention of falls.[7] Improving mobility of your spine and strength in your legs will directly improve your walking.

Of course you don't specifically need to see a physiotherapist that specialises in Pilates and neurology as they are not that easy to find, but there are many Pilates instructors out there who are updating their qualifications so that they can work confidently teaching people with specific conditions and this includes Parkinson's. Why are they doing this? Because current research and anecdotal evidence is emerging about the benefits of Pilates within rehabilitation.[8] A great combination might be regular Pilates sessions (at least weekly) with input from a physiotherapist for reassessment and monitoring. The frequency of the physiotherapist sessions would be dependent on each individual case but could be anything from monthly to yearly. A Pilates instructor with close links to a neurological physiotherapist would be ideal.

What You may Need to Work On

A Pilates programme for Parkinson's should include exercises that are going to get your spine moving especially through extension (straightening up), bending to the side and rotation (twisting). An ideal programme would also include exercises that are going to improve stability around the shoulder blades to allow free, flowing arm movements and then integrate this shoulder stability and free arm movement with spine movement. Another area to work on is hip mobility in all directions, and then integrate this into walking and balance activities, as well as any sports or activities particular to each client.[9] With Parkinson's you need to be careful that tightness in muscles that flex or bend joints don't take over, and so our programmes include more extension or stretching out exercises compared to flexing exercises. For example if your hip flexors (the muscles at the front of your hips that bend them) are tightening, the programme will include hip mobility exercises that really work on opening the hip joint up. If your hamstrings, the muscles at the back of your thighs, are getting tight and your knee can't quite fully straighten then we want to lengthen that leg and gently stretch those muscles at the back. A lot of the Pilates exercises, such as the *single leg stretch* and *dying bugs* challenge your co-ordination. As you improve with these exercises, you should notice that your co-ordination in everyday activities will also improve.

Relating the Principles of Pilates to Parkinson's

Breathing: Breathing control is a large part of Pilates and may help improve respiratory function that can decrease in Parkinson's due to postural changes. Breathing control also contributes to better core muscle activity.[10] Breathing also has the ability to relax a tense body.

Concentration: remember that during a Pilates session you should be mindful of each exercise (no writing shopping lists!) For people whose automatic control of movement is decreased, this more cognitive approach can be helpful.

Centering: The centre is the powerhouse from which the arms and legs are moved. A strong core allows your arms and legs to move more freely and improves core stability. This, and the next principle are particularly important for people developing postural changes that impact on the correct use of abdominal and back muscles, and hence affect postural control (balance).

Control: You will achieve improved muscle control and achieve better movement quality, which may help the motor symptoms experienced with Parkinson's such as slowness of movement, freedom to move limbs and a reduction in the feeling of stiffness.

Precision: We want you to aim to perform the exercises with precision leading to greater conscious and kinaesthetic control. *Kinaesthetic cueing* is when you focus on how a movement feels and how it relates to the body. Again, this precision can be very useful when automatic control is decreased.

Flowing movements: Pilates exercises are fluid, smooth and continuous. This can help with the bradykinesia (or slow movement) and decreased range of movement due to rigidity.

Two additional Principles

Isolation: Mindfulness of each exercise allows you and your instructor to recognise incorrect movements so that you can isolate the particular movement, make corrections and practice. Being mindful brings precision, which in turn increases conscious control of movement. People with Parkinson's who have been on medications for several years, and whose muscles and joints are stiffer can find it difficult to 'feel' different parts of their body to isolate the movement. This work on isolation is therefore an important part of the programme, initially requiring more assistance from the Pilates Instructor.

Routine: Pilates should form part of your weekly routine: carrying out a programme such as Pilates that incorporates flexibility and strength 3–4 times a week (as well as cardiovascular) is recommended for people with Parkinson's to sustain benefits.[11]

Cognitive and Cueing Strategies

Earlier in the book we mentioned cueing strategies and how we use these in physiotherapy to help our clients. With Parkinson's there can be disturbance of the processes in the brain that we are not conscious of (internal cueing) which affects automatic sequential movements such as walking. Physiotherapists may use cueing strategies such as visual cues like tape on the floor, or an auditory cue such as a metronome to provide a trigger or strategies to help movements. We can use cognitive strategies: for example getting the client to think about the task or movement they are trying to achieve, and breaking it up into separate components. If we use the strategies early on within the Pilates programme we may improve movement but you will be familiar with these techniques if you have to use them for other tasks such as walking. There are several cues that can help, and the three examples most pertinent to Pilates are listed below:

Mental Rehearsal

We might ask you to prepare for the task or exercise by mentally rehearsing it in your mind before you carry it out. This primes the body so it is ready to perform more effectively. You can also try it on your own during your own practice.

Visualisation

Visualisation and imagery are used a lot in Pilates to improve positioning and alignment and can be useful to Parkinson's clients who can use this technique to combat the lack of automatic control. For example when working on posture the instructor might ask you to "feel taller in your spine, imagining you have helium balloons attached to the base of the skull and tops of shoulders, gently floating you upwards."

Verbal Cues (external cue)

We will use words such as 'flowing', 'gentle', 'smoothly' which, with the visualisation can help to reduce unwanted muscle activity, and might in some cases reduce tremors, which can interfere with movement.

Summary

- Pilates is a holistic exercise technique comprising of a wide variety of exercises.
- Pilates aims to improve strength, flexibility, balance, co-ordination, correct breathing and relieve stress, which are all very important for clients with Parkinson's.
- The core principles of Pilates apply, as do two additional principles for people with Parkinson's, to enhance an exercise programme for optimal

benefits. These are concentration, breathing, centering, control, precision, flowing movements, plus isolation and routine.
- Cueing strategies can be incorporated into a Pilates programme, which might help with the loss of automatic control that clients with Parkinson's can experience. For example, visual or auditory cues and imagery.

PART TWO

In the next few chapters we are going to suggest some suitable exercise programmes. At the start of each chapter there is a brief introduction about the principles behind the exercises and how particular movements can be helpful with problems you might encounter if you have Parkinson's.

You will find a whole array of different machines in a Pilates studio. In this book we offer a few exercises that work on the areas potentially affected by Parkinson's but they are also the ones that our clients with Parkinson's particularly enjoy or find beneficial.

CHAPTER 5

Basic Pilates Exercise Programme

5 Steps of Your Routine

These exercises are designed to be performed at home on a regular basis. Don't worry if at first they seem complicated, it is difficult to control breathing, think about your deep tummy muscles and wave your arms around at the same time, but after a little practice it will all come together and you will be able to progress to slightly harder exercises. Initially you should aim to spend no more than twenty minutes on the exercises three times a week. Never do too many repetitions of one exercise: up to ten is enough, remembering that it is better to do an exercise five times perfectly rather than ten times badly.

Start with the first 5 exercises from step 1 and progress further once you feel you have understood each exercise. Begin with 5 repetitions and work up to 10 gradually. When you feel you have mastered these exercises add a couple more from each category on different days. For instance one day you could add some pelvic stabilisation exercises (Step 2), another day add upper back work (Step 3) and another day add rotation and spine stretching (Step 4). If you have any of the props at home you can build those exercises into your routine too.

Always finish your exercise session with some gentle stretches from Step 5 and try to practice the ankle and foot exercises (Step 6) as often as you can by getting into the habit of circling your ankles or stretching your calves whenever you have a spare moment. This is very important for people with Parkinson's, as stiff feet and ankles will contribute to balance and mobility problems.

Always try to vary your exercise regime as then you are challenging your mind as well as your body.

Try to exercise three times a week and continue to add and change your routine as you progress remembering to keep the variety of the different categories, always finishing with Step 5 – the stretches.

A. Take note of important 'Tips'.

B. All the exercises are gentle and safe but note any possible areas that could be problematic, or are not advised (contra-indications), grey.

C. Some of the exercises may cause discomfort, which is entirely natural. But if the experience is of an actual pain, then leave the exercise out of your programme until you have seen the Pilates Instructor. If it is more of a discomfort and unpleasant, perhaps try it again in another week or so. Sometimes, a stiff body that has not moved or been stretched for a while can signal discomfort, but it is actually a movement you need to be doing to get the part moving and more flexible ready to strengthen it up.

Breathing and Deep Core Muscles

Breathing Exercises

Breathing exercises or breathing control requires you to be very mindful of your breathing pattern so it will involve cognitive strategies or 'thinking'. This breathing technique is used throughout the Pilates exercises. It is really important that we breathe properly although, in reality, many of us don't.

Try this breathing exercise: Sit comfortably on a chair or on the bed, resting your back against the back of the chair (or on pillows if you are sitting up on the bed). If you are on a chair make sure your feet are firmly on the ground, if they aren't, place them on a large book or thick telephone directory. Put your hands gently on your tummy just under your rib cage. Breathe in slowly through your nose and feel the air go down to the bottom of your ribs. You should expand gently to the sides of the lower ribcage and your tummy should rise a little but not puff out. Feel the gentle movement under your hands. Now breathe out through your mouth. The out-breath should be ideally longer than the in-breathe, but for those people with Parkinson's whose ribcage is stiff, you want to also concentrate on a long in-breath as well. On the out-breath, feel your shoulders drop as the tension leaves them. You can also do your breathing exercises in the Pilates rest position, lying on the floor.

When we are feeling breathless or can't quite catch our breath, it is tempting to concentrate on the in-breath in an effort to take in as much air as possible. But remember the out-breath is just as important to empty our lungs sufficiently of the air that has already been used so we are ready for the next intake of oxygen rich air. If you do the breathing exercises as we describe, gently expanding the lateral tummy area and rib cage, you will breathe more effectively, taking in more air to the bases of the lungs. Puffing out our upper chests like a sergeant major is less efficient and doesn't use all the lung tissue available. Do about five of these gentle, relaxing breaths, but don't do too many in one go as you might start to feel a little faint. As you relax you may feel positive effects on any rigidity or tremor as muscles can 'let go'. Don't worry if the tremor actually seems to worsen. Sometimes, the stiffness at shoulders and upper arms hides a tremor, so when these upper arm muscles are relaxed, the tremor can become less inhibited. The breathing will also assist your potential to improve aerobic capacity; especially if the joints of your thoracic cage and spine have become stiff. A correct technique for the out-breath can stimulate better core stability as an important core muscle, transversus abdominus, is activated when you control your breath out. All this will have a positive effect on your postural control.

Exercises for the Abdominal Muscles and Pelvis

All Pilates exercises require mindfulness and cognitive strategies in order to perform them correctly. Good breathing control is required throughout to enhance relaxation, thoracic and spine mobility and core stability. As you learn these exercises you will feel how they strengthen you.

Selected abdominal exercises ensure that joints throughout your spine are mobilised with rotation incorporated, especially important in people with Parkinson's experiencing decreased spinal movement. The strength and mobility achieved with these exercises will improve balance and posture. The pelvic tilts mobilise and stabilise the pelvis, which will provide you with a strong base from which your legs can move. This will hopefully carry over into other activities such as walking or standing tasks where you need to transfer your weight from side to side. When you go from a sitting to standing position your pelvis needs to smoothly and subtly change position throughout the movement. If this subtle movement doesn't occur you will find everyday movements such as getting in and out of bed or up from a chair quite difficult.

As with most Pilates exercises there are a few different movements going on during one exercise, for example the large pelvic tilts with arms. As you practice these you will find you become more co-ordinated and you will soon realise you can't just *do* the exercises but you have to *feel* them as well.

Lie on your back with yours knees bent and hip width apart.

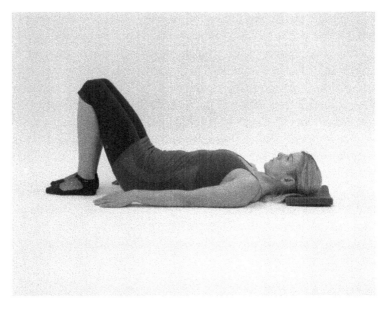

Figure 16. Pilates rest position.

Feel that you have a natural curve in the spine (neutral spine) and that the two hipbones are on the same horizontal plane as your pubic bone. Shoulders and ribcage should be relaxed with a feeling that your shoulder blades are sliding down your back with your arms down by your side.

Step 1: Breathing and Deep Core Muscles (exercises 1–9)

1 Breathing
Technique

- Lie on your back in the rest position with your knees bent and your feet hip width apart. Support your head with a small cushion. Relax your ribcage and feel the natural curve in your spine.
- Place your hands on your tummy, breathe in through the nose expanding the ribcage laterally (think of filling the sides of the ribcage with air but keep the abdominal muscles relaxed). Breathe out through the mouth holding the pelvis still.

2 Deep Transverse (lateral) Abdominal Muscles
Technique

- Your starting position is as for exercise 1.
- Breathe in through the nose expanding the ribcage laterally.
- Breathe out through the mouth drawing in with the deep lateral tummy muscles.

Tip

Imagine you are tightening a girdle around your pelvis or pulling the hip-bones towards each other as you exhale.

3 Pelvic Floor
Technique

- Repeat exercise 2 but on the exhale tighten the internal sling of muscles running from the coccyx at the base of the spine, towards the pubic bone and lift upwards through the torso.
- Try to connect the bottom of the front of the ribcage with the pubic bone as well as pulling the two hipbones towards each other making sure there is no movement in the pelvis.
- Relax completely between each repetition.

Tip

Imagine you are tightening and lifting an internal pelvic structure which is supporting the organs within your pelvis. Once you have mastered this exercise you can do it standing or sitting and try to feel that you are lifting and supporting the organs of the pelvic girdle against gravity.

4 Pelvic curls (Pelvic floor and deep abdominals)
Avoid if you have osteoporosis as this exercise can put too much pressure on the vertebrae.
Technique

- In the rest position, place your arms by your side with the palms facing down.
- Breathe in through the nose expanding the ribcage laterally.

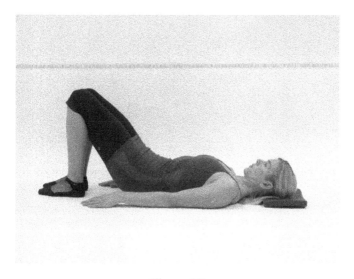

Figure 17

- Breathe out through the mouth drawing up with the pelvic floor and deep lateral abdominal muscles and curl the tailbone up just slightly off the floor.

Tips

- Be careful not to shorten the torso.
- Try to keep the distance between the ribcage and hipbones the same throughout.
- Imagine you are hollowing out the tummy and allowing the lumbar spine to stretch as you perform the pelvic curl.

5 Larger Pelvic Curls

Avoid if you have osteoporosis as too much pressure can be placed on the vertebrae.

Technique

- Start in the rest position. Breathe in through the nose expanding the ribcage laterally.
- Breathe out through the mouth drawing up with the pelvic floor and deep lateral abdominal muscles and curl the tailbone off the floor, then keep peeling the tailbone higher one vertebrae at a time until you reach a bridge position.
- Take a breath in at the top.

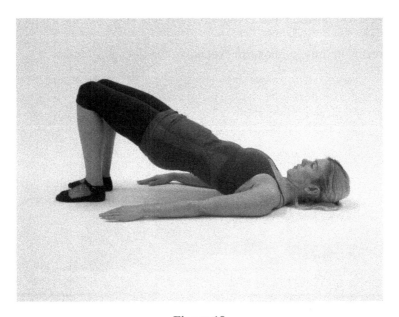

Figure 18

- Breathe out whilst curling back down through the spine using the abdominal muscles to guide the pelvis down one vertebra at a time.
- Be careful not to go up too high into the bridge causing the back to arch.

Tips

Think of the tail bone leading on the way up–but slowing the pelvis (like a brake) on the way down.

6 Arm Circles
Technique

- Start in the rest position with your arms by your side and the palms facing down.
- Breathe in through the nose taking the arms up to the ceiling.
- Breathe out placing the shoulder blades on the floor and stretch the arms behind your head drawing the bottom of the ribcage down towards your hipbones.
- Take another breath in, breathe out as you draw your shoulder blades down and circle the arms round the side and back to your hips.

Tips

- As you stretch back go as far as you can without lifting the ribcage or arching the back.
- As you circle the arms back to the starting position relax the elbows slightly and draw the shoulder blades down away from the ears.

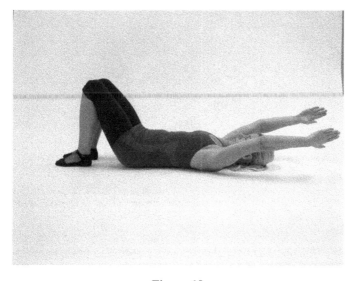

Figure 19

- Imagine your arms are wings attached to your spine and controlled by the back muscles.

7 Pelvic Curls With Arm Circles (exercises 5 and 6 together)

If you have osteoporosis avoid this exercise as too much pressure can be placed on the vertebrae and continue with arm circles as for *exercise 6*.

Technique

- Breathe in to prepare.
- Breathe out whilst drawing up with pelvic floor and deep lateral abdominal muscles then curl the tailbone off the floor until you reach a bridge position.
- Inhale, taking the arms up to the ceiling.
- Breathe out and curl back down through the spine using the tummy muscles to guide the pelvis down one vertebra at a time whilst reaching up to the ceiling with the finger tips.
- Take a breath in, as you breathe out place the shoulder blades back on the floor and stretch the arms behind your head.
- Take another breath in, breathe out as you circle the arms around the side and back to your hips.

Tips

- As you stretch back go as far as you can go without lifting the ribcage or arching the back.

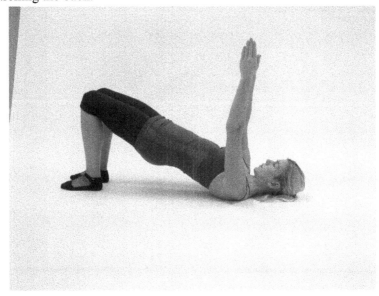

Figure 20

- As you circle the arms back to the starting position relax the elbows slightly and draw the shoulder blades down away from the ears.
- As you stretch your arms behind you and back to the starting position imagine you are having an enormous and very relaxed yawn.

8 Chest lifts

Avoid this exercise if you have osteoporosis as there may be increased pressure on the vertebrae.

Avoid this exercise if you have a problem with your neck as it may become aggravated.

Technique

- Lie on your back in the rest position with your knees bent and feet hip width apart.
- Support your head with a small cushion.
- Place your hands behind your head with the fingers linked, thumbs running down behind your ears and elbows out to the side (just within your peripheral vision).
- Breathe in and drop the chin slightly towards the chest.
- Breathe out and draw in the deep abdominal muscles and lift the upper body off the floor.
- Breathe in to return to the starting position.

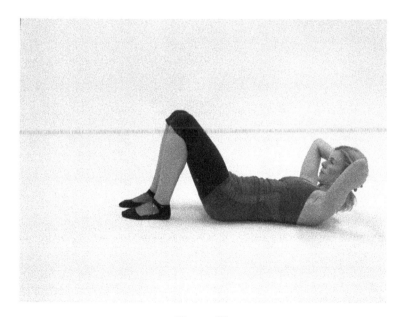

Figure 21

Tips

- Try not to let the pelvis move at all during the lift.
- Think of lifting the chest rather than pulling the head up.
- Try to maintain a stable pelvis – imagine it is strapped to the floor and only your upper body is able to move.

9 Oblique Chest Lifts

Avoid this exercise if you have osteoporosis as there may be increased pressure on the vertebrae.

Avoid this exercise if you have a problem with your neck as it may become aggravated.

Technique

- Lie on your back in the rest position with the feet hip width apart.
- Support your head with a small cushion.
- Place your right hand behind your neck with the left arm resting across your body.
- Breathe in and drop the chin slightly towards the chest.
- Breathe out, draw in the deep abdominal muscles and lift the upper body off the floor while slightly rotating to the right and reaching the left arm towards the right knee.
- Breathe in to return to starting position.
- Repeat 5 times and then to the other side.

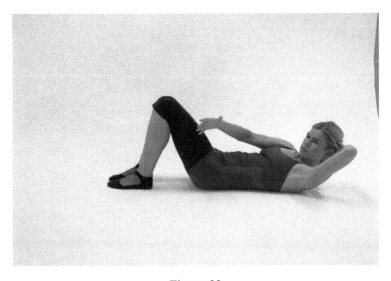

Figure 22

Tips
- Keep the reaching arm soft.
- Think of rotating both shoulders as you lift, you are not rolling onto one.
- Don't let the opposite hip lift up off the mat.

Try to maintain a stable pelvis – imagine it is strapped to the floor and only your upper body is able to move.

Step 2: Pelvic Stabilisation (exercises 10–16)

Leg Slides and Dying Bugs, Four Point Swimming

Exercises such as these are great for strengthening the core at the same time as moving your arms and legs together; the legs stretch out one at a time so your hamstrings are really lengthened. A lot of concentration and co-ordination are required and all this at the same time as breathing correctly!! As you become more advanced at Pilates and really feel how individual exercises work on several different areas simultaneously you may notice improvement in your dual tasking ability.

The concentration required will encourage you to be more mindful as you work on co-ordination, strength and flexibility. This exercise should also make you laugh and bring out your inner child!

10 Leg slides and dying bugs
Technique
- Start in the rest position.

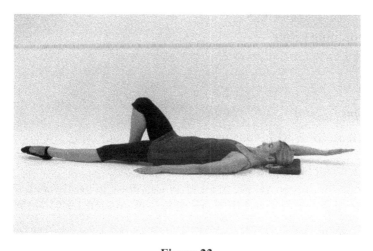

Figure 23

- Breathe in and take one arm up to ceiling.
- Breathe out and take the arm behind your head towards the floor as the opposite foot slides along the mat until the leg is fully stretched out.
- Inhale and return the leg to the starting position and arm up to ceiling.

Tips
- Reach to the end of your figure tips but only take the arm as far as possible without lifting your ribcage or arching your back.
- Make sure your pelvis remains still when bringing the straight leg back to the starting position.
- Repeat on the opposite side.
- You can leave the arms out of the exercises to begin with, just stretching the legs out one at a time (leg slides).
- Imagine your deep abdominal muscles are the control centre for your limbs.

Prone Exercises

By prone we mean lying on your tummy. You are working on core strength, joint mobility, co-ordination, dual tasking and reaching. But also in this position you are stretching out muscles that might get tight and lead to more flexion, which can happen with Parkinson's. The exercises work the extensor muscles of the back and inhibit the flexor muscles and fibres of upper trapezius, which will allow you to maintain a better posture.

This is an excellent position for people with Parkinson's to work in, but do not go into this position if you have a stiff neck or shoulders, or if your hip flexors will not stretch and cause back and hip pain. Wait until you have seen the Pilates Instructor to ensure you will not injure yourself actually getting into, but more importantly getting back out of the position.

11 Swimming prone

Avoid this exercise if you have a condition of the spine called spondylolisthesis (slipping of vertebra) as it can be made worse.

Technique
- Lie face down with your legs straight and your arms stretched up by your ears.
- Place a soft book or towel under your forehead.
- Breathe in to prepare, breathe out as you draw in gently with the deep abdominal muscles and lift your right arm and left leg slightly off the floor.
- Breathe in to return to starting position.
- Breathe out and repeat on other side.

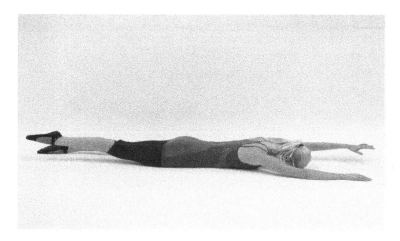

Figure 24

Tips

- Place a pillow under your tummy if you feel discomfort in your lower back.
- Don't expect to lift the arm or leg very high off the ground.
- Try to keep the shoulders drawn down your back.
- Try not to lift the hip of the working leg.
- Lengthen the limbs at the start of the exercise then just lift them up away from the floor.

12 Four point swimming
Technique

- Start on all fours, your hips should be over the knees and your shoulders over your hands.

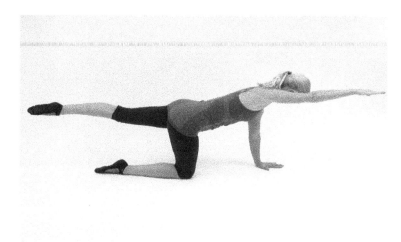

Figure 25

- Breathe in to prepare, breathe out as you draw in with the deep abdominal muscles and lift right arm and left leg slightly off the floor.
- Breathe in to return to the starting position.
- Breathe out and repeat on the other side.

Tips
- Think of sliding the foot along the floor before it lifts.
- Hold the torso still while keeping the tummy muscles engaged throughout.
- Don't take the leg or arm too high, your lower back should not arch.
- Keep the back of the neck long (don't lift the chin).

Knee Drops, Clam and Scissors

In these exercises you continue to do your mindful breathing. You are gently drawing in your deep tummy muscles to maintain a stable core but now you are moving one limb (leg). The trick is to keep good alignment and stability around your centre as you work on strength and mobility of a single limb with good movement control.

13 Knee Drops
Technique

- Lie on your back in the rest position with your knees bent and feet hip width apart.
- Support your head with a small cushion.
- Breathe in and allow one knee to open to the side, about 45 degrees.

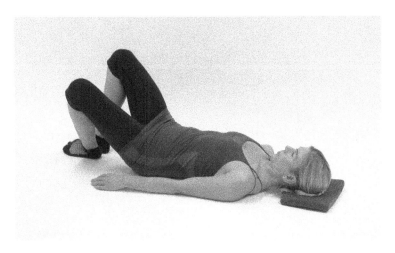

Figure 26

- Breathe out and bring it back to the starting position.
- Repeat 5 times with each leg.

Tips
- Don't let the opposite hip lift as you open the knee.
- Keep the abdominal muscles engaged.
- Try placing your hands on the hipbones to help hold the pelvis still as you open the knee.

14 Clam (Alternative to Knee drops)
Technique

- Lie on your side (preferably against a wall).
- Support your head with a cushion and place a rolled up towel under your waist to support the gentle curve of your waist.
- Have your hips and knees bent at about a 60-degree angle with your feet in line with your spine.
- Breathe in to prepare, breathe out, draw in with the deep abdominal muscles and lift the top knee towards the ceiling keeping the feet together and without moving the pelvis.
- Breathe in and place the knee back to starting position.

Tips
- Try not to sink into the towel with your waist. Think of lifting away from the towel with the tummy muscles and this will help to hold the hips still.
- Try not to rock the top hip backwards.
- Think of a clam and the opening hinge movement initiating from the deep buttock muscles.

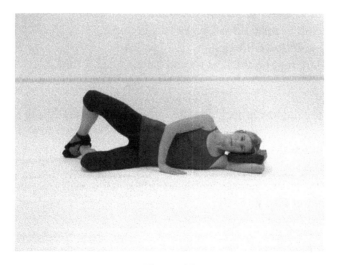

Figure 27

15 Knee Lifts (Scissors)

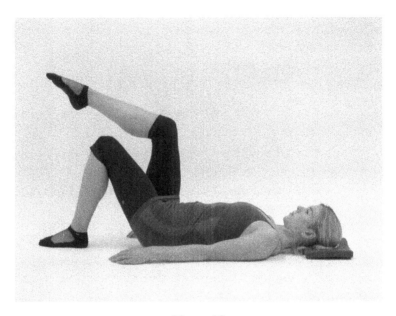

Figure 28

Technique

- Lie on your back in the rest position.
- Support your head with a small cushion.
- Breathe in to prepare, breathe out, draw in the deep tummy muscles and float the knee up to tabletop (where your hip and knee are at 90 degrees).
- Breath in to lower it back to the starting position.
- Breathe out to raise the other leg to tabletop.
- Breathe in to lower the leg.
- Repeat, alternating the legs so you lift each leg 5 times.

Tips

- Make sure the lower back does not arch when you are lifting or lowering the legs.
- Try to move the legs from the hips only without any movement in the pelvis at all.

16 Side Lying Hip Exercise
Technique

- Lie on your side (preferably against a wall).
- Support your head with a cushion and place a rolled up towel under your waist.

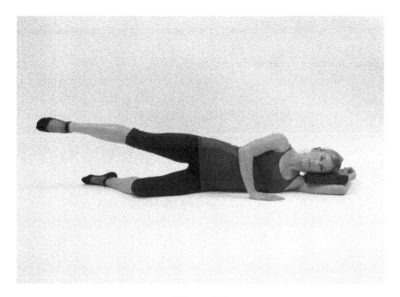

Figure 29

- Bend the bottom leg, keep the top leg straight with the foot slightly flexed (the toes are pulled forward).
- Breathe in to prepare, breathe out, draw in with the deep tummy muscles and lift the top leg towards the ceiling without moving the pelvis.
- Breathe in and lower the leg.

Tips

- Make sure the knee faces forward – don't let it turn up to the ceiling as you lift the leg.
- Place your hand on the outside of your thigh and initiate the movement by pushing up against your hand.

Step 3: Exercises for the Upper Back (exercises 17–20)

Shoulder Stabilisation

These exercises are often done as a set with the *dumb waiter*, usually sitting on a stool with the feet firmly on the ground. The arm extensions will work on scapula stability and gently open up the front of the chest. In this exercise we are trying to relax the upper fibres of trapezius and instead engage the lower fibres as well as working latissimus dorsi, which extends the arms behind us.

17 Shoulder Stabilisation
Technique

- Start seated on a chair or balance ball.
- Make sure your knees are aligned and level with your hips (place a book under your feet if necessary to keep the knees at right angles with hips).
- Have your arms down by the side (you can hold light weights or baked bean cans if you wish too).
- Breathe in and shrug the shoulders up to the ears.
- Breathe out and lower them down whilst drawing in with the deep abdominal muscles.
- Breathe in and rotate the arms so that the palms face back.
- Breathe out as you draw the shoulders blades down and move the arms slightly behind your torso initiating the movement from below the shoulder blades.
- Breathe in and return the arms to the starting position.

Tips

- Make sure that shoulders do not roll forward as arms move behind body.
- Try not to let the ribcage flare.
- Keep the abdominals pulled in and the torso still – only the arms should move.

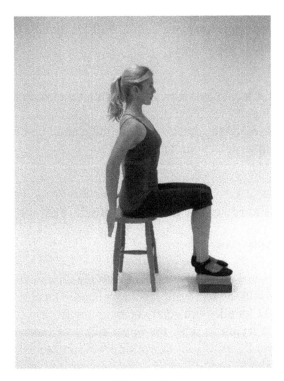

Figure 30

- Keep the back of the neck long.
- Don't squeeze the shoulders back – it is a very gentle movement.
- Imagine the arms swinging gently back and forth like a pendulum without any movement in the torso.

18 Dumb Waiter

Technique

- Start seated on a chair or balance ball.
- Make sure knees are aligned and level with hips (place a book under the feet if necessary to keep the knees at right angles with hips).
- Start with arms bent and your elbows gently held into the waist. Your palms should be facing in with fingers long.
- Breathe in to prepare, breathe out and rotate the arms to the side.
- Breathe in to return the arms to the starting position.

Tips

- Keep the elbows still – do not allow them to move behind body.
- Don't lock the elbows into your waist.
- Sit up tall with the abdominal muscles activated.

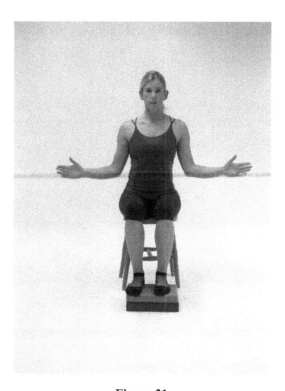

Figure 31

19 Prone Arrow with elbows bent

Avoid if you have a painful degenerative neck condition, such as spondylo-listhesis or advanced arthritis, or if your neck is so stiff with the Parkinson's you cannot get into this position without help.

Technique

- Lie face down with your legs straight and hands palms down by your shoulders with elbows pointing up to the ceiling.
- Place a cushion or soft book under your forehead.
- Breathe in to prepare, breathe out as you draw in with the deep abdominal muscles, lengthen the tailbone towards your feet and push the elbows down to the floor.
- Once you feel the shoulder blades pulling down lift the upper back and head keeping the chin down towards your chest.
- Breathe in to return to starting position.

Tips

- Place a pillow under your tummy if you feel discomfort in your lower back, or under your hips if they are initially too tight to stretch fully.
- Don't lift the shoulders and head too far off the floor.
- Keep the chin down stretching the back of the neck.
- The neck should stay long at the back, in line with your spine. Imagine that you have a glass of water balancing on your neck that you don't want to spill.

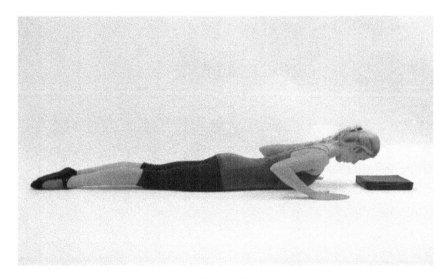

Figure 32

20 Diamond Press

Avoid if you have a painful degenerative neck condition, such as spondylo-listhesis or advanced arthritis, or if your neck is so stiff with the Parkinson's that you cannot get into this position without help.

Technique

- Lie face down with your legs straight, your arms should be bent and your hands in a diamond shape under your forehead with the thumb and forefingers touching.
- Breathe in to prepare, breathe out as you draw in with the deep abdominal muscles and lengthen the tailbone towards the feet. Press gently down onto your forearms lifting the upper back and head off the floor.
- Breathe in and return to starting position.

Tips

- Place a pillow under your tummy if you feel discomfort in your lower back or under your hips if they are initially too tight to stretch fully.
- Don't lift the shoulders and head too far off the floor.
- Keep the neck in line with the spine (keep chin down).
- Draw the shoulder blades down as you press into the floor with the forearms.
- Feel your upper torso lifting off the floor whilst the rest of body remains still.

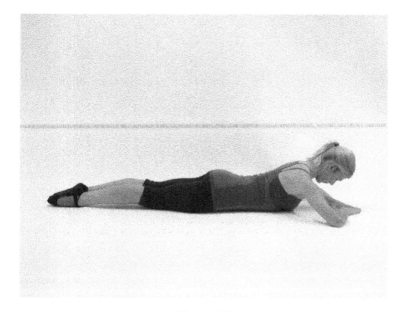

Figure 33

Step 4: Rotate and Stretch the Spine (exercises 21–25)

These exercises work on shoulder and thoracic spine mobility, which will loosen up the joints and hopefully allow more arm swing and thoracic rotation during walking. We mentioned in previous chapters how trunk rotation and arm swing can be reduced with Parkinson's so it's really important to keep these joints moving. During these exercises, not only will you be working on movement of the joints but also stability of the surrounding area, particularly the shoulder blades or scapulae and the core so that you have a firm base from which to move.

21 Cossack Arms

Avoid if you have osteoporosis as the rotation may cause increased pressure on the vertebrae.

Technique

- Start seated on a chair or balance ball.
- Make sure knees are aligned and level with hips (place a book under feet if necessary).

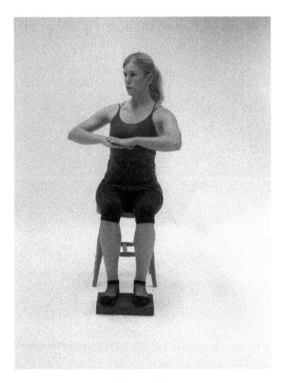

Figure 34

- Place one hand on top of other in front of chest with elbows held out to side.
- Breathe in to prepare, breathe out as you draw the abdominal muscles in and rotate the upper body to one side.
- Breathe in to return to centre.
- Breathe out and repeat to other side.

Tips

- Try to keep the shoulders down and hands in middle of chest bone.
- Try to keep the pelvis still and knees facing forward.
- Imagine your spine is a straight rod and your torso a square box rotating around it. Imagine your hips and knees have headlights on them that need to keep facing forwards.

22 The Cat

Be careful if you have osteoporosis as too much flexion may cause increased pressure on the vertebrae. Instead just go from flat back to arched back (avoiding angry cat).

Technique

- Start on all fours with the hips over knees and your shoulders over the hands.
- Breathe in to prepare, breathe out as you draw the deep abdominal muscles in – drop the head so you are looking between the knees. Your

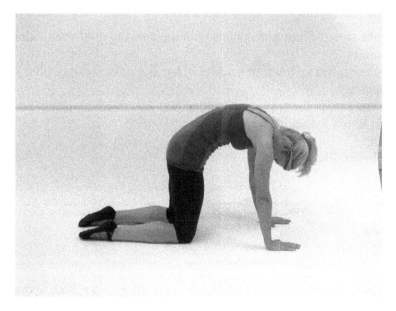

Figure 35

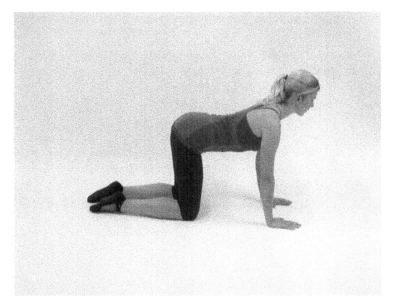

Figure 36

tailbone should tuck under and draw down so that the back is arched like an angry cat.
- Breathe in to come back to a flat back.
- Breathe out and arch the other way so that you are looking up and sticking your bottom out – a happy cat!

Tips

- Make sure the movement starts with the drawing in of your abdominal muscles.
- Place a rolled up towel under heel of hands to take pressure off wrists if necessary.
- When you do the angry cat position feel the stretch all along the spine and across the shoulder blades.

23 Thread The Needle

Avoid if you have osteoporosis as the flexion and rotation and may cause increased pressure on the vertebrae.

Technique

- Start on all fours with your hips over the knees and shoulders over the hands.
- Breathe in to prepare, breathe out as you draw in the deep abdominal muscles and reach with one hand under the opposite arm in the direction of the hip.

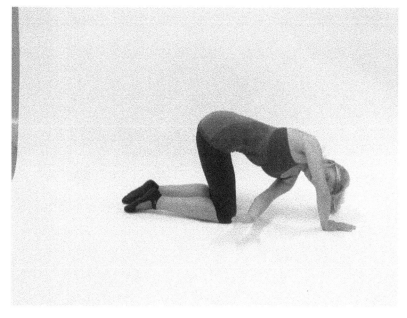

Figure 37

- Breathe in as you bring the arm back and stretch it up to the ceiling.

Tips

- Allow the shoulder of the moving arm to drop towards the floor.
- Keep the neck relaxed following the direction of the moving arm.
- Think of the arm threading through the hole of the needle and feel the stretch around the shoulder blade.

24 Round The World Stretch

Avoid if you have osteoporosis as the rotation may cause increased pressure on the vertebrae.

Technique

- Lie on your side with head supported by a cushion and hips and knees bent.
- Both arms should be outstretched in front of you on the floor, palm to palm.
- Breathe in and take the top arm up to ceiling, breathe out and take the arm all the way over to try to touch floor behind you.
- Hold the stretch for 2 breaths.
- Breathe in and lift the arm back to ceiling.

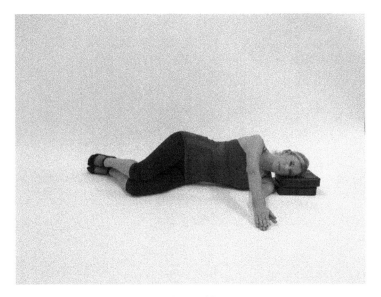

Figure 38

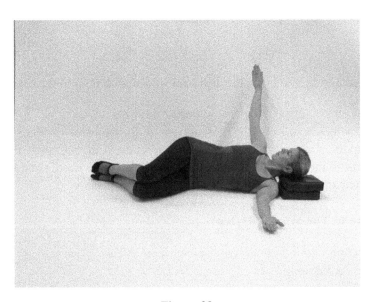

Figure 39

- Breathe out and place the hand back on other palm.

Tips

- Follow the arm with your head.
- Keep the shoulders relaxed and breathe into the stretch.
- You should get a lovely opening feeling across the chest and shoulders during this exercise.

25 Windmills

Technique

- Lie on your back in the rest position.
- Have a tightly rolled up towel width ways, under the shoulder blades.
- Breathe in and take both arms up to the ceiling, breathe out and scissor your arms – one back towards your ear and the other towards your hip.

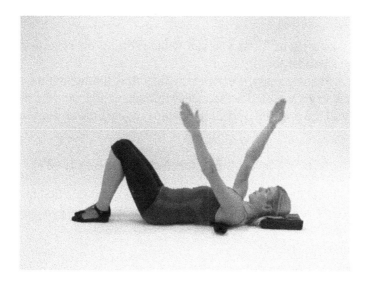

Figure 40

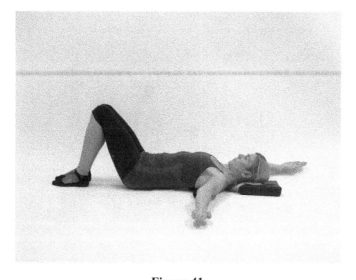

Figure 41

- Breathe in and return both arms to the ceiling.
- Breathe out and scissor the arms the other way.
- Breathe in and return to ceiling.
- Breathe out and scissor again then continue around like a windmill taking the top arm down to hip and bottom arm up to ear.
- Breathe in and return the arms to the ceiling.
- Repeat, alternating the direction of the windmill.
- Keep the abdominal muscles engaged so as not to arch the lower back.

Tips

- Only take arms as far as you can without lifting the ribcage or feeling pain in shoulder joint.
- Keep reaching out to the ends of the fingertips throughout the exercise.
- Don't worry if you find the sequence difficult to pick up – the main thing is to hold the position of the torso whilst moving the arms around.

Step 5: Stretching Exercises (exercises 26–31)

A gentle stretching programme will encourage relaxation and muscle and joint mobility so be sure to allow good time at the end of your session.

26 Hamstring Stretch
Technique

- Lie on your back.
- Place a theraband (or any length of material) around one foot and hold the ends.

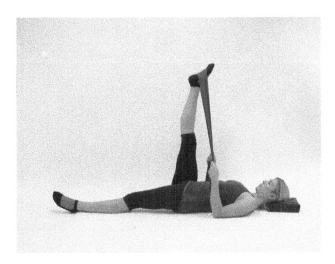

Figure 42

• Lift the foot to the ceiling gently stretching hamstrings (back of leg).

Tips

• Try to keep the tailbone from lifting off the floor.
• Bend other knee if any discomfort is felt in lower back.

27 Sitting Hamstring Stretch

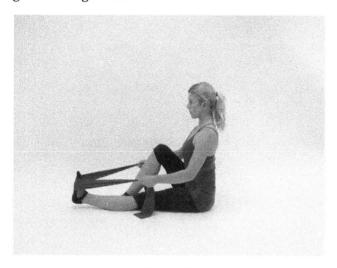

Figure 43

Technique

• Sit up straight with one leg outstretched in front and the other bent up with the knee dropped out to the side.
• Place the band over the toes of outstretched foot and hold the ends.
• Pull the toes towards you with the band feeling the stretch through the calf and back of knee.

Tips

• Try to sit up as tall and straight as possible.

28 Lower Back (lumbar) Stretch
Technique

• Lie on your back and lift your legs with the knees bent, holding your knees with your hands.
• Breathe in to prepare, breathe out and gently pull one knee towards the chest.
• Breathe in to return.
• Breathe out to pull the other knee towards the chest.
• Breathe in to return.

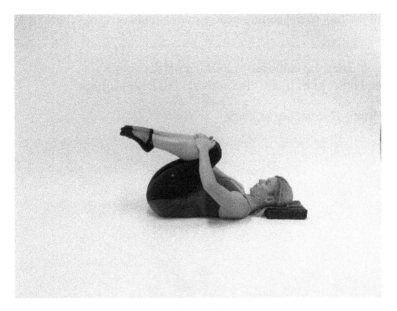

Figure 44

- Breathe out and gently pull both knees towards your chest and feel the stretch in your lumbar spine.

29 Large Hip Rolls

Avoid if you have osteoporosis as the rotation may cause increased pressure on the vertebrae.

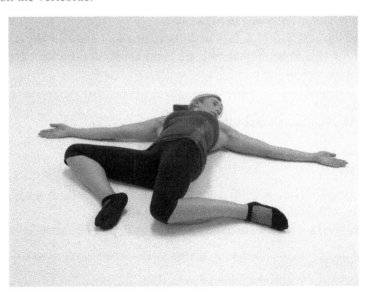

Figure 45

Technique

- Lie on your back with the knees bent and feet hip width apart.
- Have your arms stretched out to the side.
- Breathe in to prepare then breathe out and take both knees over to one side turning the head in the opposite direction.
- Hold the stretch for a few breaths.
- Breathe in, breathe out and take the knees all the way over to the opposite side changing the direction of the head.

Tips

- Lift the bottom foot and place on the top knee for extra stretch.

30 Side Stretch – seated
Technique

- Sit sideways on a chair with the arm nearest to back of chair above your head and the other arm across your waist holding onto the back of the chair.
- Breathe in to prepare, breathe out and reach away from the back of the chair with stretched arm.

Tips

- Try to keep the torso as long as possible.
- Turn your head over the shoulder in the direction of stretch.

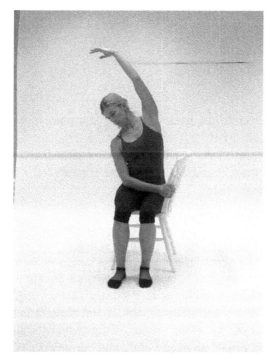

Figure 46

- Remember to do both sides.

31 Calf Stretch

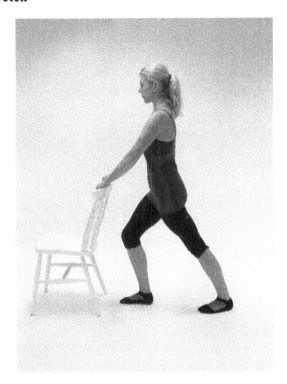

Figure 47

Technique

- Stand holding onto the back of a chair and place one foot behind the other, hip width apart.
- Breathe in to prepare, as you breathe out bend the forward knee, keeping the back leg straight and the heel on the ground.
- Repeat on the other leg.

Step 6: Foot Work

We have added a few foot exercises, as it is not uncommon for us to see people with Parkinson's who have very stiff feet and tight ankles. If we get good range of movement in our ankles and more mobility in our feet it will hopefully allow increased sensory information to be sent effectively to our central nervous system and brain and our balance will be improved.

So don't forget your feet!! You can even buy small spikey balls to roll your foot around on to increase the sensation further.

Ankles

Ankle Mobilisers

- Circle the ankle 10 times in each direction. Then pull the foot up and point down 10 times.
- Repeat with the other side.

Ankle Stretches

- Stand on the bottom step of your stairs with the heels hanging off the back.
- Go up onto the balls of your feet, then slowly lower your heels down so they are lower than the step and feel the stretch on the back of your calves.
- Repeat 3–4 times.

Footwork

Do these exercises standing, gently holding a chair or wall in front, or sitting with your feet firmly on the ground. You can do feet together or separately.

Toe Exercises

Try and lift the big toe up without the other toes, then relax. This is often an easy exercise as people with Parkinson's begin to use the big toe to help raise the foot when walking as the ankle muscle weakens or stiffens. It is therefore also important to exercise the toe into a downward position. So stretch the big toe downwards, curling it towards the sole of the foot, and then relax.

Now try and lift up the other toes without the big toe.

This is a mind over matter exercises and will suddenly "click".

Try this exercises whilst you are in the bath with your feet resting either side of the taps.

Towel Exercise

Place a towel under the very ends of your toes. Try and draw the towel towards your heel without your toes "clawing". If the toes do claw then stop and start again.

CHAPTER 6

Add Some Props

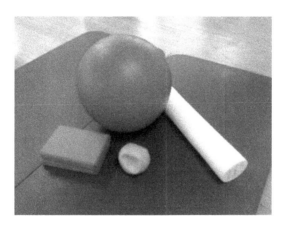

Figure 48

Any exercise can be adapted or enhanced using props such as the foam roller, exercise band, small inflatable ball (18cm diameter) or large gym ball (normally 55–65cm diameter).

The foam roller comes in different lengths and diameters but we suggest a 90cm length with a 15cm diameter. This is a full roller but if your balance isn't great you may want to start with a half roller. Exercise band comes in different strengths depending on what you are trying to achieve. We advise using a medium strength to start with. The gym ball is large and very strong. The diameter you need depends on your height but the two most common sizes are 55cm for a person of height 4'8" to 5'5" and 65cm for height 5'6" to 6'0".

When using props the possibilities are endless and we have only offered a few ideas to start with. You can get any of the items for reasonable prices from a sports shop or well-stocked large supermarket, or on the Internet. Most can be tidied away except perhaps the gym ball!

Take note of the neck exercises, which can be done with small inflatable ball under the base of the head. These will include rotation and working the muscles at the front of the neck known as the deep neck flexors, which are important for stability and good neck posture. Good neck mobility and posture is important for many movements and daily activities and allows improved visual input, which is really important for balance. If we have good neck posture we are less prone to pain in this region.

With Parkinson's, the mid back or thoracic spine can become bent forwards and to compensate for this the neck has to tip backwards at its base to lift the head up. The pectoral muscles at the front of the shoulder can also get tight. It is really important to address this issue to avoid discomfort. The foam rollers are great to get your thoracic spine extending and an exercise such as *chicken wings* will give your pectorals a really good stretch.

Small Inflatable Ball

For exercises 1–3 lie on your back in the rest position with a slightly inflated small ball under your neck.

Place a cushion under knees for comfort if desired.

1 Deep Neck Flexors

Breathe in to prepare, breathe out and draw you chin down a little towards your chest about 1 or 2 inches or until you feel a gentle lengthening at the back of your neck.

Breathe in to relax.

Imagine you have a ripe, soft peach under your chin. You want to hold it there but not so firmly that you bruise it or break the skin.

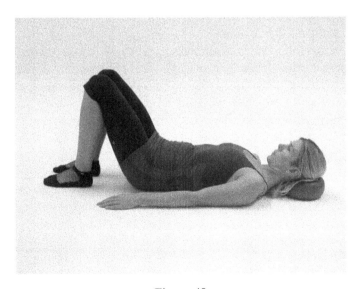

Figure 49

2 Neck Rotation
Technique

- Keep the small ball under your neck and your chin gently drawn down, holding the imaginary soft peach.
- Breathe in to prepare, breathe out and turn the head to one side.
- Breathe in to come back to the middle.
- Breathe out to turn to the other side.
- Breathe in to come back to the middle.

Tips

- Keep the soft peach held in the same position under your chin through the exercise.

3 Neck Relaxer
Technique

- Start in the rest position with the ball under your neck.
- Breathe deeply to relax.
- Make very small figures of 8 with your nose until you feel the neck muscles relax.

Tips

- After about 5, go in the opposite direction.
- This exercise is more effective and relaxing if performed with your eyes closed.
- Drop the chin to gently stretch the neck extensor muscles.
- You can try drawing circles with your nose; keep them to the size of a 10 pence piece.

Gym (or balance) Ball

1 Low Abdominal Strengthening
Technique

- Lie on your back with your ankles on the ball and legs straight.
- Hold the spine and pelvis in neutral (keeping a natural curve in your spine).
- Breathe in to prepare, breathe out and draw in the pelvic floor and deep abdominals whilst bending the knees towards you.
- Breathe in and return the legs to a straightened position.

Tips

- Make sure you don't allow the pelvis to move (keep the natural curve of the spine) as the legs bend.

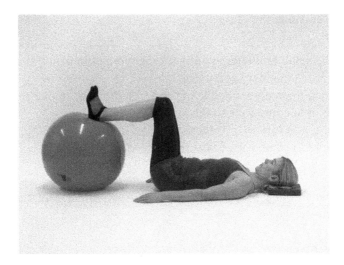

Figure 50

- Add a little resistance to the legs as they move.

Imagine it is the low abdominals that are drawing the knees in towards you.

2 Bridge

Avoid if you have osteoporosis as too much pressure can be placed on the vertebrae.

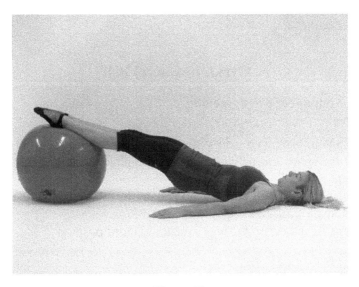

Figure 51

Technique

- Lie on your back with legs straight, this time have your and calves on the ball.
- Your arms should be outstretched by your side with the palms down.
- Breathe in to prepare, breathe out and engage the deep abdominals and buttock muscles as you lift the torso up off the floor coming up onto your shoulder blades.
- Breathe in and return to starting position.

Tip

- Do not go too high off the floor: you shouldn't feel any discomfort in the lower back.

3 Hip rolls

Avoid if you have osteoporosis as the rotation may put too much pressure on the spine.

Technique

- Lie on your back with your legs over the ball. Your hips and knees should be bent to 90 degrees.
- Breathe in to prepare, breathe out as you draw in the abdominals and gently roll the knees over to one side.
- Breathe in, breathe out and roll the knees over to other side.

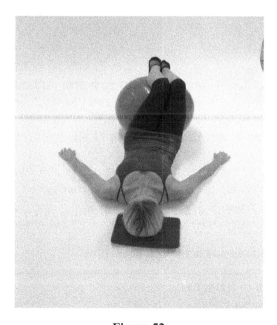

Figure 52

Tips

- Don't let the hip come up too high at first.
- Don't twist the pelvis just roll the knees from side to side.

4 Back stretch

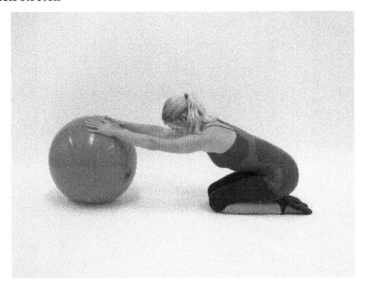

Figure 53

Avoid if you have osteoporosis as the flexion can put too much pressure on the spine.

Technique

- Kneel on the floor sitting back onto your feet. Try placing a cushion under the feet or between your bottom and your feet if uncomfortable.
- Alternatively, sit on a low stool if you are unable to kneel.
- Place your hands onto the ball in front of you with your fingers facing upwards.
- Breathe in to prepare, breathe out and push the ball away as far as possible whilst keeping the bottom back on the heels.
- Breathe in to return.

Tip

- Try to keep the spine curved and head down.

5 Back Stretch to Diagonal

Avoid if you have osteoporosis as the flexion can put too much pressure on the spine.

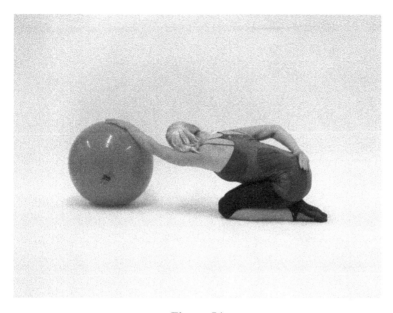

Figure 54

Technique

- Kneel on the floor sitting back onto your feet. Try placing a cushion under the feet or between your bottom and your feet if uncomfortable.
- Alternatively, sit on a low stool if you are unable to kneel.
- Place one hand on the ball with fingers facing upwards and the other arm behind your Back.
- Breathe in to prepare, breathe out and push the ball away across your body whilst keeping the seated position.
- Breathe in to return.
- Repeat to the other side.

Tip

- Try to keep the spine curved and head down.

Foam Roller

For exercises 1–3 you should lie on the roller so that it is the length of the spine but also supporting the head. Have your knees bent and the feet on the floor, slightly apart. Make sure spine and pelvis are in neutral (keep the natural curve of spine).

1 Fly
Technique

- Breathe in and take both arms up to the ceiling with palms facing in.

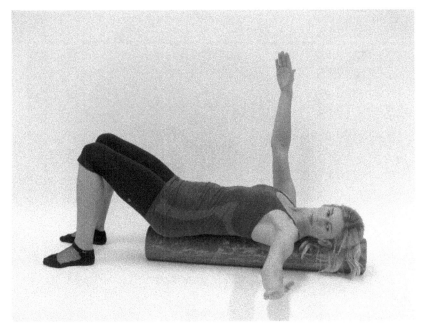

Figure 60

- Breathe out and take one arm to the side turning the head to follow the hand.
- Breathe in and return the arm to the starting position.
- Breathe out and repeat to other side.
- Take the feet a little closer towards each other each time (if possible) to challenge your core strength.
- Make sure the knees stay over the toes.
- Don't arch the lower back during the exercise.

2 Dying Bugs
Technique

- Take one arm up to the ceiling with the palm facing forward and opposite leg up to table top (hip and knee bent at right angles).
- Breathe in to prepare, breathe out, engage the deep abdominals and take the arm back towards ear and stretch the leg out straight with the hip at an angle of 45 degrees (so that the knees are approximately level).
- Breathe in and return to the starting position.
- Repeat 5 times and then change to the other leg and arm.

Tips

- Do not drop the leg too low.

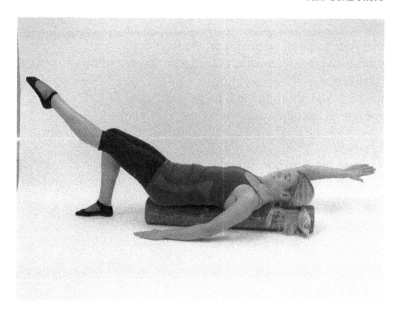

Figure 61

• Only take arm as far back as possible without lifting rib cage.

3 Leg Lifts

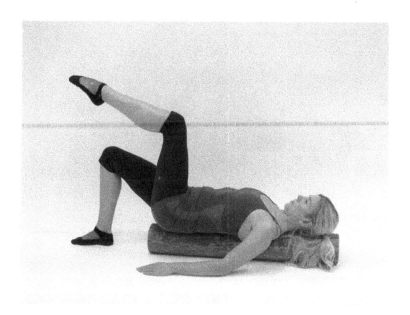

Figure 62

Technique

- Have your hands by your side on the floor.
- Breath in to prepare, breathe out, engage the abdominals and lift one leg to tabletop.
- Breathe in and return the foot to the floor.
- Repeat with the other side.

Tips

- Try to use the deep core muscles without moving pelvis.
- Try to put a little pressure through heel of supporting leg to help stabilise the pelvis.

4 Swan
Technique

- Lie on your tummy with the arms outstretched, the forearms on the roller and the palms facing inwards.
- Breathe in to prepare, breathe out, engage the lower abdominals and lengthen your tailbone towards your feet.
- Draw the shoulder blades down and slightly lift the upper body as the roller moves towards your wrists.
- Breathe in to return to starting position.

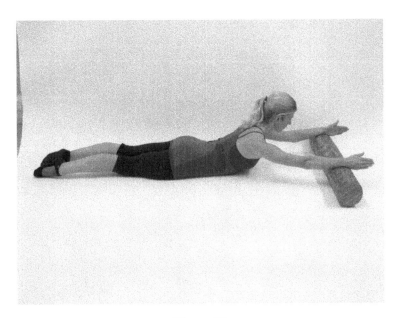

Figure 64

Tips

- Don't lift upper body too high.
- There shouldn't be any discomfort in lumbar spine.
- Keep the neck in line with the spine – don't lift the chin.

5 Chicken Wings
Technique

- Lie on roller so that it is the length of the spine and the head is supported. Have the knees bent and the feet hip width apart.
- Breathe in and take arms to the ceiling, breathe out and take the arms behind the head.
- Breathe in, breathe out and take the arms out to the side, bending your elbows and shoulders into right angle positions parallel to floor.
- Hold the stretch for a few breaths.
- Take the arms back down by your sides.
- Then repeat.

Tips

- Be careful not to arch your back when taking the arms behind your head.
- Feel the stretch across the front of your shoulders and chest.

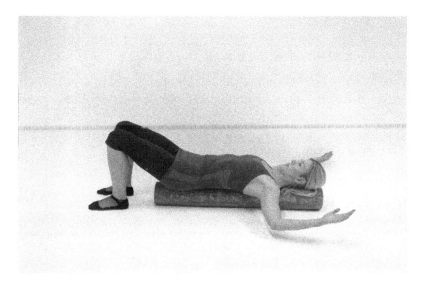

Figure 65

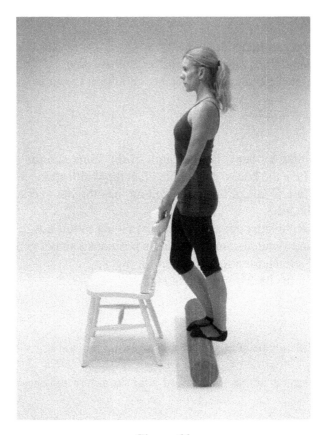

Figure 66

6 Standing Calf Stretch
Technique

- Stand on roller holding onto something stable such as a kitchen surface or high backed armchair.
- Bend one knee and allowing the heel of other foot to drop down towards floor stretching calf muscle.
- Hold for a few breaths then repeat with the other leg.

7 Neck Roll
Technique

- Lie on your back in the rest position with the knees bent and the foam roller widthways under your neck.
- Have your arms out to side gently holding the ends of the roller.
- Breathe deeply and turn the head from one side to another allowing the foam roller to gently massage the neck.

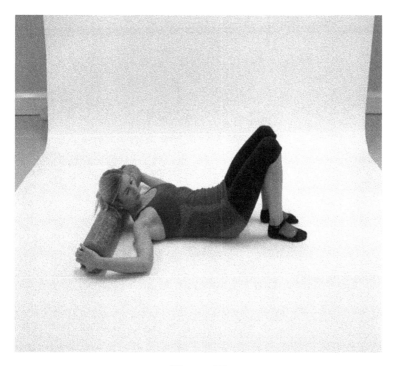

Figure 67

CHAPTER 7

Reformer Exercise Programme for Parkinson's

Joseph Pilates Universal Reformer: Designed to *"universally reform the body"*.

The Reformer was invented by Joseph Pilates when he was providing rehabilitation to soldiers on the Isle of Man during the war. He attached springs and machinery to the bedposts of hospital beds, which allowed patients to practice his Contrology exercises and strengthen muscles and joints whilst lying down.

It is the most versatile of all Pilates equipment as the exercises can be performed on your back, side, sitting or standing and even upside down. The springs can be adjusted to achieve different results and ropes are attached with stirrups to work the limbs too. Most exercises require you to either push or pull the carriage but some are performed holding it steady for control.

Because of these different dimensions there are literally hundreds of exercises that can be performed on the Reformer and all of these can then be adapted to suit individual abilities and conditions.

Using the Reformer not only adds interest and fun to the exercises but also, using the resistance and support of the springs, allows you to improve flexibility and balance, lengthen and strengthen muscles and achieve far greater results than just doing mat work exercises.

It has a moveable carriage, an adjustable foot bar and shoulder rests (usually removable) and 5 springs of 3 different colours:

Green – heavy
Red – medium
Bluc – light
Yellow – very light

On each exercise we will suggest the springs to be used but this is really down to the Pilates instructor's decision and varies with the weight and ability of the client. There is also a box that comes with the Reformer,

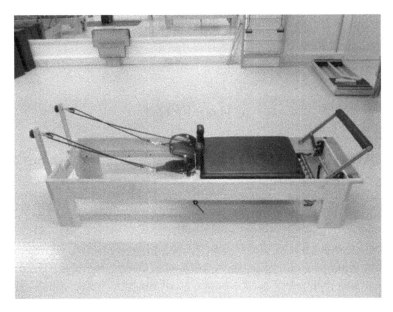

Figure 68. Reformer machine.

which you can sit or lie on and this is used in varying positions for many of the exercises.

These exercises should only be performed under the guidance of a Pilates instructor with the required qualification.

Leg Work

These exercises are designed to mobilise and strengthen the hip and knee joints whilst maintaining a stable pelvis. Adjust the carriage position to avoid over flexing the knee joints or hip joints (your instructor can show you how to do this).

1 Parallel Legs

1 blue and 1 red spring or 2 red springs

Technique

- Lie on the reformer with the arch of your feet on the foot bar.
- Have your legs hip width apart.
- Make sure your spine is in neutral i.e. with a natural curve of the spine and your pelvis is in neutral.
- Breathe in to prepare, breathe out, engage your deep abdominal muscles and push away from the bar straightening your legs.
- Breathe in to return to the starting position.

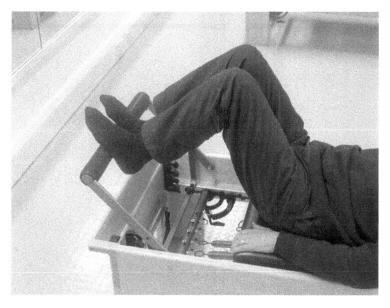

Figure 69

Tips

- Make sure you don't move the pelvis (lift the tail bone) as you push away from the bar.
- Try not to push the shoulders up against the shoulder rests.
- Try to feel that you are gliding back and forth with your pelvis strong, good flowing movement through your knee and hip joints, ribcage and shoulders should stay completely relaxed.

2 Single Leg Parallel

1 red spring or 1 blue | 1 red

Technique

- Lie on the reformer with the arch of your foot on the foot bar.
- Bend the other leg to table top and support the knee with your hand.
- Make sure your spine is in neutral.
- Breathe in to prepare, breathe out engaging the deep abdominal muscles and push away from the bar straightening your leg.
- Breathe in to return to starting position.

Tips

- Make sure you don't move the pelvis as you push away from the bar.
- Try not to push the shoulders up against the shoulder rests.

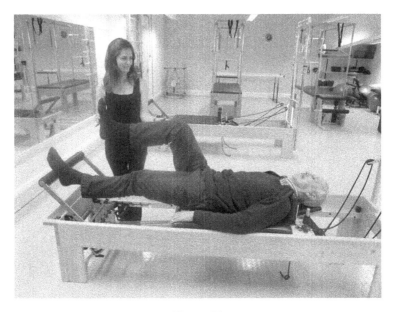

Figure 70

- This is a good exercise for balancing out leg strength – try to do 5 repetitions on your weaker side, 5 on your stronger side and then repeat 5 again on the weak side. Increase the repetitions as necessary.

3 Wide V Position With Rotation

1 blue and 1 red – or 2 red springs

Start with your knees bent, your heels wide apart on the foot bar and externally rotate the legs from the hips.

Technique

- Make sure your spine is in neutral.
- Engage your deep abdominal muscles and push away from the bar straightening your legs.
- Keeping the legs as straight as possible rotate your legs inward, swivelling on your heels.
- Return to the foot bar bending the knees towards each other.
- Push out again straightening the legs with the knees facing inwards.
- Rotate your legs outward swivelling on your heels.
- Bend the knees outwards and return to the foot bar.

Tips

- Keep the breathing relaxed and rhythmical throughout the exercise.
- Try to lift up with your core muscles as you rotate within the hip joints.
- Gently swivel on your heels rather than push on the bar.

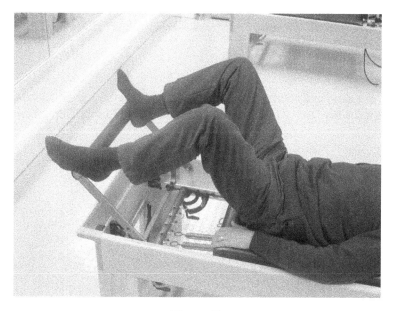

Figure 71

- Make sure you maintain neutral spine throughout.
- This exercise is a wonderful hip mobiliser – visualise the ball and socket joints of the hip and feel you are creating an easy movement in and out.

4 Prancers

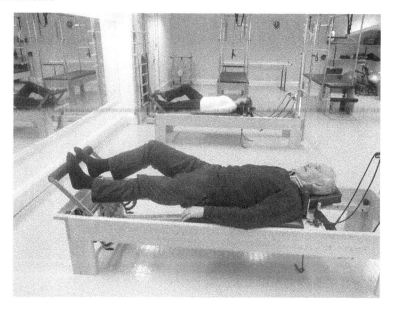

Figure 72

1 blue and red or 2 red springs

Place the toes parallel on the foot bar parallel and hip width apart.

Technique

- Breathe in and push away from the bar so that both your legs are straight.
- Breathe out and bend one knee keeping both feet on the bar and allow the opposite heel to fall under the bar stretching the calf muscles and tendons.
- Breathe in to straighten.
- Alternate several times.

Tips

- Keep the breathing relaxed and rhythmical throughout the exercise.
- This is a very good non weight-bearing stretch for the Achilles tendons which can become very tight and affect your walking pattern.

5 Leg Work With Board

Place the jump board onto the end of the Reformer (your instructor will show you how).

1 blue and 1 red spring or 2 red springs

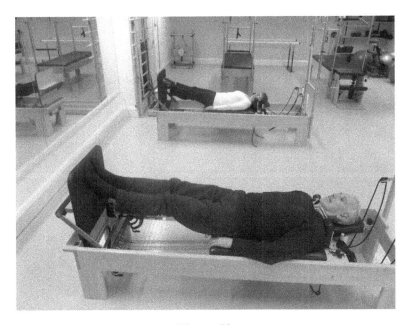

Figure 73

Technique

- Lie on your back with your feet on the board.
- Have your knees bent with legs parallel and hip width apart.
- Allow your heels to lift as much as needed.
- Engage your deep abdominal muscles and push away from the board until the legs are straight and the heels are in contact with the board.
- Now, lift your heels away from the board maintaining contact with your toe joints (as if standing on tiptoes) and keep the legs straight.
- Lower your heels back onto the board then slowly bend the knees and return to the starting position allowing your heels to lift off when needed.

Tips

- Keep the breathing relaxed and rhythmical throughout the exercise.
- Try to use the core muscles to move the carriage throughout (don't just push into the feet).
- Feel the movement through the ankles and toe joints now – as well as the hips and knees.

6 Single Leg Work With Board

Place the jump board onto the end of the Reformer.

1 Blue or 1 red spring

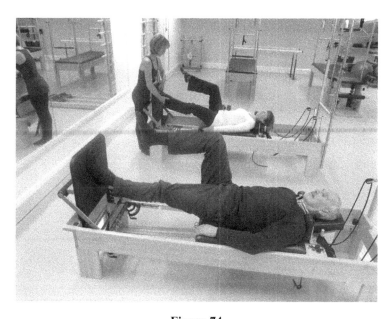

Figure 74

Technique

- Lie on your back with one foot on the board and knee bent.
- Other leg is bent to tabletop with the knee supported by your hand.
- Engage your deep abdominal muscles and push away from the board until the leg is straight and the heel is lowered.
- Lift your heel away from the board maintaining contact with your toe joints and keeping the leg straight.
- Lower your heel back onto the board then slowly bend the knee and return to the starting position lifting your heel when needed.

Tips

- Keep the breathing relaxed and rhythmical throughout the exercise.
- Remember to use the core muscles to move the carriage throughout (don't just push into the foot).
- Don't do too many repetitions in one go and be aware of alignment. The hip, knee and toes should all be in line with each other.
- Adjust the repetitions to increase strength or mobility on one leg.

7 Side Lying Hip Flexion

1 red and 1 blue spring

Technique

- Lie on your side in the middle of the carriage with your head supported by a pillow.
- Place your top foot along the bar slightly in front of your torso with the leg bent.
- Bend the other leg comfortably underneath you.

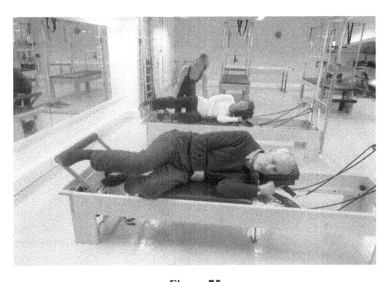

Figure 75

- Breathe in to prepare then breathe out and push away from the bar straightening the leg.
- Breathe in and lift the heel off the bar then lower it back down keeping the leg straight.
- Breathe out and slowly return to the bent position keeping the knee at the same level as the hip.

Tips

- Try to maintain hip and knee alignment throughout.
- Make sure the bar is set at the same height as your hip.
- Do not drop into your waist – keep a little gap under your waist or put a rolled up towel under there and "lift away" from it.
- Imagine your top leg is resting on a glass coffee table to maintain good alignment without dropping down or lifting off.

8 Side Lying Hip Flexion (in extension)

1 red and 1 blue spring

Technique

- Lie on your side in the middle of the carriage with your head supported by a pillow.
- Place your top foot along the bar but this time slightly behind your torso with the leg bent and heel lifted.

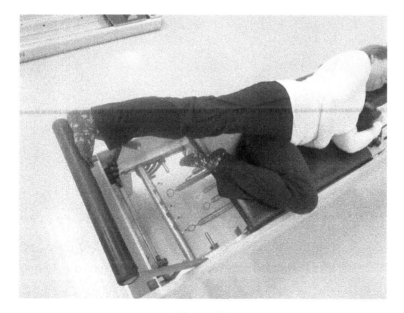

Figure 76

- Bend the other leg comfortably underneath you.
- Breathe in to prepare, breathe out and push away from the bar straightening the leg and lowering the heel.
- Breathe in, breathe out and slowly return to the bent position keeping the knee at the same level as the hip.

Tips

- Try to keep the top hip forward – don't let it be pulled back by the leg.
- Maintain neutral spine don't let the back arch as the leg straightens.
- Do not drop into your waist – keep a little gap under your waist using a rolled up towel if necessary.

This exercise can help with mobility to widen your stride when walking.

9 Hip Circles

1 blue and 1 red or 2 red springs

Technique

- Lie with feet in stirrups and legs straight at a 45 degrees angle (your instructor can help you into this position to begin with).
- Holding the pelvis still, circle the legs down and around in a circle from the hip joints.
- Repeat up to 10 times, then change direction this time going up first and then back down and around.

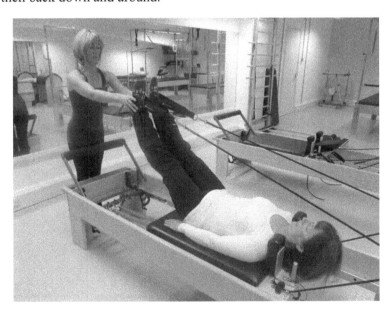

Figure 77

Tips

- Keep the breathing relaxed and rhythmical throughout the exercise.
- Keep the legs parallel (with the knees facing up to the ceiling) through-out the circle.
- Be careful not to go too high or too low with the leg: keep the circle fairly small around the 45 degree angle.
- Try to lead with the toes and reach out with long legs but without lock-ing the knees.
- Hold the torso still and feel that you are mobilising the hip joints only.
- Try to visualise the ball and socket joint of the hip moving through its range of movement.

10 Hip Circles With External Rotation

1 blue and 1 red or 2 red springs

Technique

- Lie with your feet in the stirrups and your legs straight at a 45 degrees angle externally rotated from the hip joints.
- Holding the pelvis still and the legs turned out circle the legs down and around in a circle from the hip joints.
- Repeat up to 10 times then change direction and start by going up, then around.

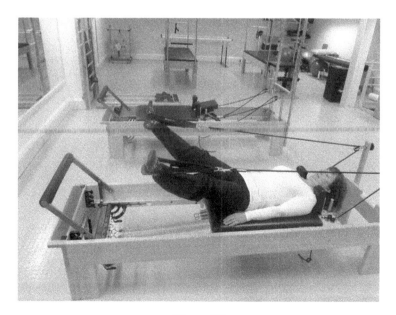

Figure 78

- Keep the breathing relaxed and rhythmical throughout the exercise.
- Keep the legs rotated outwards throughout: feel the inner thighs working hard to bring the legs together and stretching when they are apart.
- Be careful not to go too high or too low – just circle around the 45 degree angle of the hips.

Tips

- Remember to try to lead with the toes reaching out with long legs but without locking the knees.
- Hold the torso still: you are mobilising the hip joints only.
- Try to visualise the ball and socket joint of the hip moving through its range.

11 Hamstring Stretch

1 red and 1 blue spring

Technique

- Place one foot on the foot bar and straighten the leg.
- Place a stirrup on the heel of the other foot and straighten the leg.
- Allow the carriage to move by bending the leg on the bar and increasing the stretch through the hamstrings.
- Breathe into the stretch and hold for a good few minutes trying to gradually increase the stretch.
- Repeat on the other leg with the other stirrup.

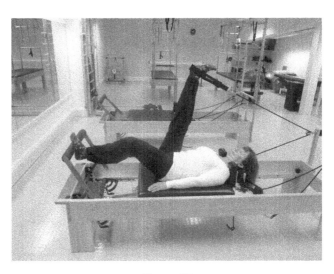

Figure 79

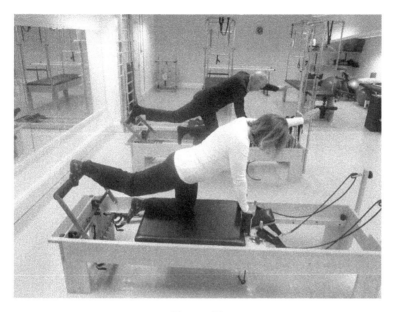

Figure 80

12 4 Point Kneeling One Arm Lifted

1 red spring

Technique

- Kneel on the reformer facing away from bar.
- Place the right hand on the shoulder rest and the other loose by your side.
- Lift the right knee and place the foot behind on the foot bar.
- Breathe in to prepare.
- Breathe out and push away from the bar straightening the leg and keeping the pelvis level whilst lifting the left arm straight out in front of you until it is level with your head.
- Breathe in whilst bending the knee to return the carriage to the starting position and lowering the arm.

Tips

- Remember not to over extend or lock the supporting elbow or lift the shoulder of the raised arm.
- Keep the deep abdominal muscles engaged throughout.
- Think of the whole of the torso remaining still and the limbs moving independently.
- Don't worry if you can't straighten the moving leg completely it is more important to keep the pelvis still.

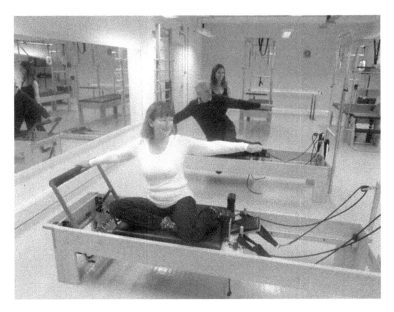

Figure 81

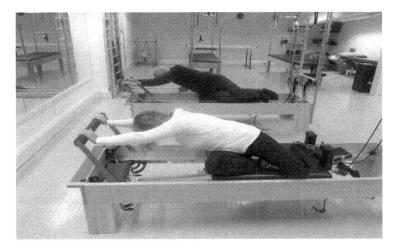

Figure 82

13 Mermaid

Avoid this exercise if you have osteoporosis as there may be increased pressure on the vertebrae. If you have painful knees, perhaps due to arthritis then you may find this exercise uncomfortable, in which case leave out or ask your instructor for adaptations or an alternative.

1 blue spring

Technique

- Kneel sideways on the reformer with the legs bent to the side towards the shoulder rests.
- Place nearest hand on the foot bar in line with the shoulder. Have the other arm relaxed by your side.
- Breathe in and push away from bar straightening the arm and extending other arm into a diagonal line. Breathe out and circle the top arm around to place onto the bar trying to get your torso parallel to the floor.
- Take a breath into this position.
- Breathe out and return to the upright starting position taking the arm back across the body letting the arm still in contact with the bar gently bend.

Tips

- Don't let the back arch during the stretch.
- Do allow the hip to lift during the stretch.
- This is a lovely rotational stretch – don't go too far too soon – just ease into the stretch.

Box on Reformer

14 Breaststroke Prep With Extension

1 red spring

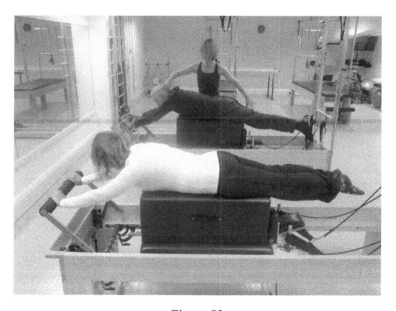

Figure 83

Technique

- Place the reformer box long ways on the carriage.
- Lie face down on the box facing the bar.
- Your hand should be resting on the bar, your elbows facing out to the side with long fingers.
- Breathe in to prepare, breathe out and draw the shoulders down – push back away from the bar lengthening the arms and swivelling the hands so that they straighten.
- Breathe in, breathe out and lift the head and shoulders up into a slight back bend.
- Breathe in to bring the head and shoulders back down to flat.
- Breathe out and open the elbows returning to the bar.

Tips

- Keep the shoulders pulled down throughout.
- Keep abdominals, buttocks and back of legs engaged on back extension to protect the lower back.
- Try to keep the head in line with the spine (don't lift the chin too high or let the head drop).
- During the back extension think of lifting the head and shoulders out of the water keeping a lovely long spine.

CHAPTER 8

Trapeze Exercise Programme for Parkinson's

The trapeze table is a versatile piece of Pilates equipment on which a variety of exercises can be performed. It uses springs attached to metal poles, which then work against gravity, and the exercises range from simple stretching to advanced acrobatics.

For the Parkinson's programme we will be concentrating on spring assisted and resisted exercises to isolate and strengthen certain muscle groups and those, which will help to stretch and rotate the body.

There are a variety of different bars and attachments used in the exercises:

- A metal push through bar at one end.
- Two springs attached to a wooden pole called the roll down bar.
- A padded trapeze bar attached to springs.
- Various attachments for different length springs on the poles.
- Single stirrups, double stirrups and handles.

The springs come in different tensions to help or challenge the client:

Short springs:

Yellow = very light
Blue – light
Red = medium

Long springs:

Yellow = light
Purple = heavy

When using the springs on the push through bar it is best to also attach the safety strap to avoid injury if the bar is let go unintentionally.

These exercises should only be performed under the guidance of a Pilates instructor with the required qualification.

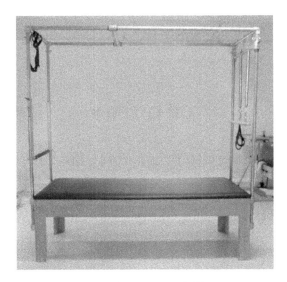

Figure 84. Trapeze Table.

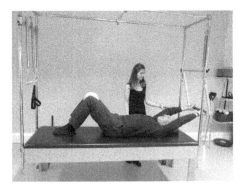

Figure 85. Push Through Bar (no springs).

1 Push Through Bar

Technique

- Start lying on your back, have your knees bent and hip width apart with a cushion between them. Hold the push through bar above your head.
- Take a breath in and bring the bar down towards your face opening the elbows out to the side, breathe out and holding neutral spine push the bar behind your head.
- Breathe in and bring the bar back to your nose.
- Breathe out and straighten your arms pushing the bar up towards the ceiling.

Tips

- Be careful not to flare (lift) the ribcage during the push through.
- Concentrate on holding the torso stable whilst moving the arms.
- This can also be performed on a foam roller for extra stretch through the chest.

2 Push Through with Inner Thigh Squeeze

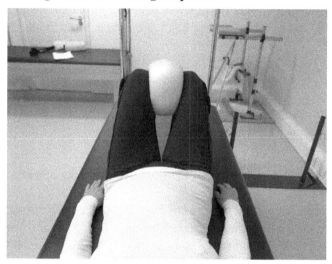

Figure 86

Technique

- Push through bar no springs.
- Start by lying on your back, knees bent hip width apart.
- Place a small bolster or Pilates ring between your thighs.
- Hold the push through bar above your head.
- Take a breath in and bring the bar down towards your face opening the elbows out to the side, breathe out and holding neutral spine push the bar behind your head whilst drawing the knees together.
- Breathe in relax the legs and bring the bar back to your nose.
- Breathe out and straighten your arms pushing the bar up towards the ceiling whilst drawing the knees together.

Tips

- Be careful not to flare (lift) the ribcage during the push through.
- Make sure that the pelvis stays in neutral throughout.
- Try to feel that the inner thigh squeeze is coming from the pelvic floor and drawing the knees together – rather than pushing the knees against the resistance using the outer thighs.

3 Mini Curl Up

Avoid this exercise if you have osteoporosis as there may be increased pressure on the vertebrae.

Technique

- Push through bar – can be done with 1 light spring attached to high hook (plus safety strap) or without springs.
- Start by lying on your back, knees bent hip width apart with a cushion between them and both arms holding the push through bar above your head.
- Take a breath in and bring the bar down towards your face opening the elbows, breathe out and holding neutral spine push the bar behind your head.
- Breathe in and bring the bar back to your nose, breathe out straighten the arms, lift your head and perform a small curl up.

Tips

- Make sure you hold the pelvis still whilst lifting the upper body in the curl up.
- Be careful not to flare (lift) the ribcage during the push through.
- On the curl up imagine you are making a C curve with your body – bringing the arms and upper body up level to the knees whilst the pelvis stays in contact with the bed.

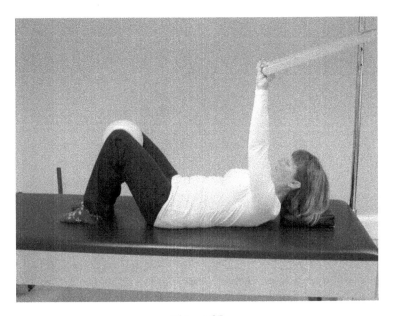

Figure 87

4 Mini Oblique Curl Ups

Avoid this exercise if you have osteoporosis as there may be increased pressure on the vertebrae.

Technique

- Push through bar – can be done with 1 light spring attached to high hook (plus safety strap) or without springs.
- Start lying on your back, knees bent hip width apart with a cushion between them. Have one arm holding the push through bar above your head and the other supporting your neck.
- Breathe in to prepare, breathe out and curl up whilst rotating towards your bent elbow outwards.
- Breathe in to return keeping arm straight.

Tips

- Be careful not to just rotate onto your shoulder – make sure you add some lift of the upper body too.
- Keep the pelvis stabilised – don't let the opposite hip lift during the rotation.
- Imagine you are making the shape of a bow and arrow with your arms as you curl up – keeping the chest open.

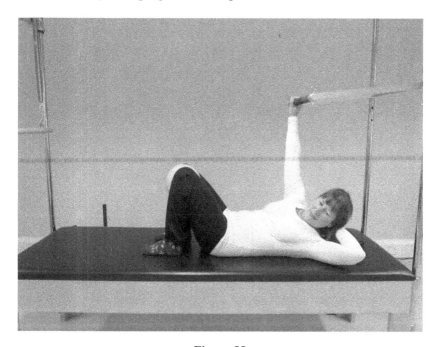

Figure 88

5 Bridge Lift With Trapeze Bar

Avoid this exercise if you have osteoporosis as there may be increased pressure on the vertebrae.

Technique

- Curl down bar with 2 long yellow springs and trapeze bar.
- Start lying on your back holding the curl down bar above your head.
- Place the trapeze bar approximately above your knees and then put your ankles into the strap with your legs straight and slightly externally rotated from the hip joints.
- Breathe in to prepare, breathe out and lift your torso up into a bridge whilst drawing the shoulder blades down and lowering the bar towards your legs.
- Breathe in to return to the starting position.

Tips

- Make sure you use abdominals, buttocks and inner thigh muscles to lift the torso.
- Initiate the arm movement from the back: don't push with the arms or let the wrists flex.
- Try to visualise the lift coming from the strong muscles of the torso – rather than using the strength of the limbs.

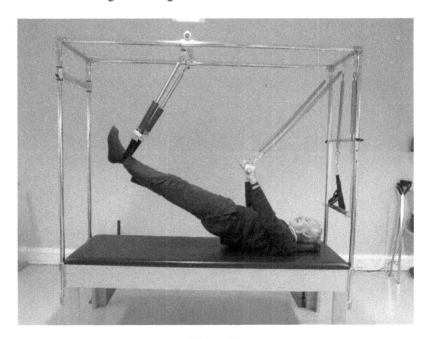

Figure 89

6 Curl Down

Avoid this exercise if you have osteoporosis as the flexion may cause increased pressure on the vertebrae.

Technique

- Curl down bar with 2 short yellow springs.
- Sit facing the curl down bar with legs straight and hip width apart.
- The arms should be at shoulder width holding the bar.
- Breathe in to prepare, breathe out, draw in the deep abdominals and start to curl through the spine until you are lying flat.
- Breathe in, breathe out, lift the chin to the chest and start to curl up through the spine.

Tips

- Articulate through the spine one vertebra at a time.
- Don't use your arms to help curl you back up.
- Don't worry if you run out of breath during the curl, just keep your breathing relaxed and regular.
- Once you have mastered this exercise you can use the longer yellow springs for more of a challenge.
- On the curl up think of the bottom of your ribcage meeting with your sitting bones to help keep flexing the spine.

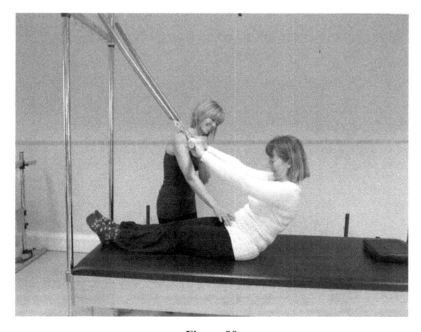

Figure 90

7 Curl Down with 4 Breaths and Rotation

Avoid this exercise if you have osteoporosis as there may be increased pressure on the vertebrae.

Technique

- Curl down bar with 2 long yellow springs.
- Sit upright with the legs straight and feet against poles.
- Hold onto the centre of the curl down bar with your left hand and have your right arm extended to front with the palm up.
- Breathe in to prepare, breathe out as you lead with your right arm and rotate upper body away from the bar.
- Take a small breath in then out and slightly curl down through the spine reaching towards the right hand.
- Take a small breath in then out and curl further touching the bed with your finger.
- Take a small breath in then out and curl further onto the bed reaching towards the pole – then roll forward onto your right hip stretching through your back and top hip.
- Breathe in, breathe out and curl back up.

Tips

- Try to keep pelvis level until the last stretch.
- Reach through the fingers with a long soft arm whilst keeping the shoulder down.
- Try to use the abdominals to curl back up (not the arm).

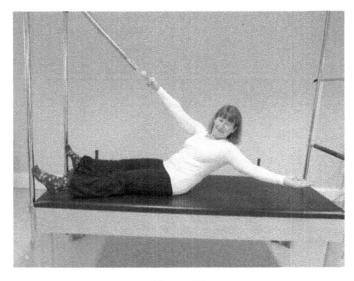

Figure 91

- Think of rotating first through the upper back and then gradually down through the length of the spine.

8 One Arm Curl Down with Side Stretch

Avoid this exercise if you have osteoporosis as there may be increased pressure on the vertebrae.

2 long yellow springs attached to 1 handle

Technique

- Sit upright with the legs straight and feet against poles.
- Hold onto the handle with your left hand and your right arm extended in front, palm facing down.
- Breathe in to prepare, breathe out and curl down through the spine until you are lying flat with your arm extended behind your head.
- Breathe in, breathe out and bend to the left side with your arm by your head also taking the right leg to touch the left (banana shape).
- Take a few breaths in this position feeling the stretch.
- When you are ready breathe out and continue to the left curling up to a sitting position.

Tips

- Remember to rotate the arm so that palm faces in on the stretch.
- Try to keep a neutral spine (don't arch the back on the stretch).
- Try to use the abdominals to curl up (not the arm).
- This is a wonderful stretch for the whole side of the body.

9 Hamstring Exercise

1 long purple spring

Technique

- Attach the spring to an appropriate height so that the resistance is comfortable.
- Lie on your back with one foot in a double stirrup attached to a long purple spring.
- Bend the knee to about a 60 degree angle and have the other knee bent as in the rest position.
- Breathe in to prepare, breathe out as you move the leg against the resistance of the spring keeping the leg the same length throughout the movement and the knee bent at the same angle.
- Breathe in and return to starting position.
- Repeat until hamstrings feel warmed and beginning to get tired.
- Then straighten the leg and gently stretch the hamstrings.

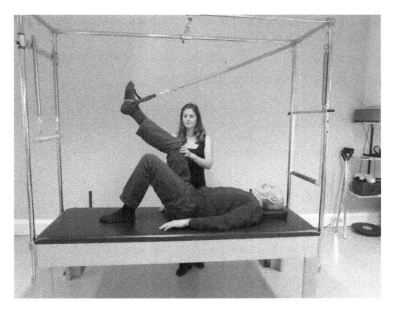

Figure 92

Tips

- The leg moves from the hip joint only.
- Do not lead with the heel.
- Keep the pelvis in neutral during the exercise and the stretch.
- Think of moving the upper part of the leg (pushing from the hamstrings) only and leading with the toes.

10 Push Through Stretch

Avoid this exercise if you have osteoporosis as there may be increased pressure on the vertebrae.

Technique

- Sit facing the push through bar with your feet against the poles and the legs straight.
- Hold the bar with both hands shoulder width apart.
- Breathe in to prepare, breathe out and push the bar forward stretching through the hamstrings and the back.
- Breathe in and return to the upright starting position.
- Breathe out and push the bar up towards the ceiling tipping forward from the pelvis and drawing the shoulder blades down.

Tips

- Keep the movement fluid.
- Don't strain the neck – keep the head in line with the spine.

11 Round the World Stretch

Avoid this exercise if you have osteoporosis as there may be increased pressure on the vertebrae.

Technique

- Sit with your feet against the poles holding the push through bar as for *exercise 10.*
- Place one hand in the centre of the bar with the other extended in front, palm facing up.
- Roll back into a pelvic curl.
- Take the extended arm around and back to make a diagonal line from fingers to opposite toes.
- Continue to take the arm behind and round into a side bend.
- Reverse all the way back around and to an upright sitting position.
- Push the bar up, rotate upper body and take hold of the opposite pole with the palm facing away from body.

Tips

- Keep the tummy muscles engaged throughout.
- Keep the pelvis in a curve whilst reaching behind (don't arch the back).
- Try to keep the movement fluid and breathe deeply through each stretch.

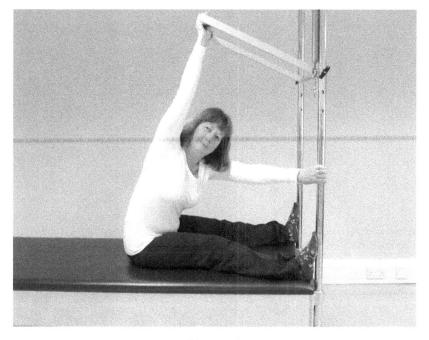

Figure 93

12 Bow and Arrow

If you have osteoporosis just to the first part of the exercise, i.e. pulling the arm back, don't add the rotation.

2 long yellow springs with handles

Stand at end of Trapeze with the long yellow springs attached to top hooks and hold handles.

Technique

- Pull one arm back bending the elbow whilst rotating to that side and allow other arm to lengthen in front.
- Return to the starting position.
- Repeat to other side.

Tips

- Keep the shoulders down throughout the exercise.
- Try to rotate from waist only.
- Stand far enough away from the machine to create resistance with the springs.
- Think of a bow and arrow and the long reach needed to fire the arrow.

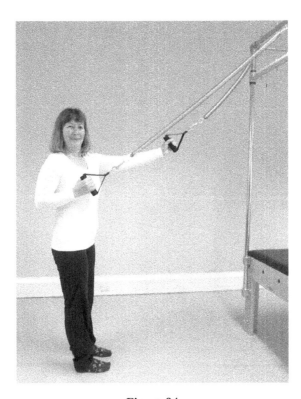

Figure 94

CHAPTER 9

Exercises for Parkinson's using The Core Align

It is essential to get up into standing and adapt exercises to this position in order to maintain or improve balance. You need to relate all the movements and techniques that you have learnt throughout the matwork exercises into functional, everyday activities such as walking. A good Pilates instructor will be able to adapt exercises to suit your needs so that you are working on the areas pertinent to you but you can also do work on the Core Align.

The Core Align is a fairly new piece of Equipment in the Pilates Studio. It is designed to challenge your core strength, balance and functional movement. It is different from the other machines as most of the exercises are performed standing therefore it is particularly good for posture and gait. Also these exercises if preferred, can be done wearing shoes (trainers).

We have included it in the Pilates for Parkinson's programme as it is necessary to improve posture and the rotational aspect of walking to avoid the shuffling gait which can develop with this condition.

The Core Align is made up of a long track with two moveable carts attached by rubber springs of varying resistance at either end. Most exercises are more demanding when done with lighter springs so change the springs to suit ability: your instructor can guide you. In addition, the moving carts will help to challenge and improve any balance or mobility issues.

There is also a ladder attached at one end and most of the exercises are performed holding onto this. Attached to the ladder are two ropes with handles which are used for some of the exercises. Keep the breathing relaxed and rhythmical throughout these exercises.

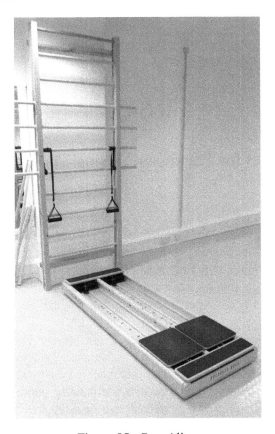

Figure 95. Core Align.

1 Morning Stretch
Technique

- Stand facing the ladder with one foot on each cart equal distance from the centre line.
- Both hands should be holding the bar at head height.
- Breathe in to prepare, on the out breath slide one foot behind whilst lunging onto the front leg.
- Allow the back heel to rise naturally.
- Breathe into the stretch then repeat on the other side.

Tips

- Keep the head facing forward in line with your spine.
- Be careful not to arch the back.
- Try to feel the gentle stretch from the shoulders right down through the back and into the calf of the extended leg – as though you are hanging from the ladder.

2 Hoof

Technique

- Stand facing the ladder holding on at waist height.
- Have one foot on each cart equal distance from the centre line.
- Bend one knee sliding the cart back and lifting the heel
- Return the leg to the starting position trying not to shift your weight from one leg to the other.
- Alternate legs.

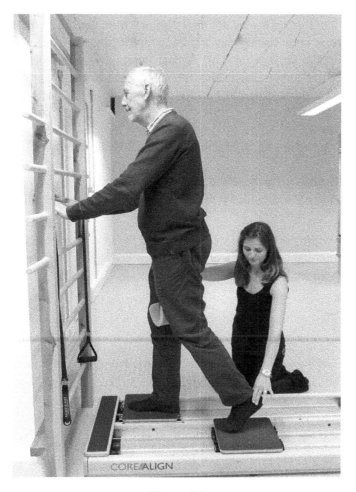

Figure 96

Tips

- Keep the knees in alignment only the lower part of the leg should move.
- Keep the spine in neutral and the pelvis still.
- Place a cushion between the thighs to help stabilise the pelvis.
- Think of showing the heel to the back of the room each time the foot glides backwards. Imagine there is a metal rod going through your knees, keeping them still so you are only moving the lower leg.

3 Hoof Window Wipe
Technique

- Stand facing the ladder holding on at waist height.
- Have one foot on each cart equal distance from the centre line.
- Bend one knee sliding the cart back and lifting the heel. At the same time lift the opposite arm off the bar, rotate the upper body in the opposite direction whilst circling the arm up and around.
- Return to the starting position trying not to shift your weight from one leg to the other.
- Alternate sides.
- Keep the knees in alignment only the lower part of the leg should move.
- Place a cushion between the thighs to help stabilise the pelvis.
- Try to keep the shoulder stabilised as the arm circles around.

Tips
Think of wiping a window with your hand to achieve the right shape and follow your hand with your head. Remember the imaginary rod going through your knees.

4 Statue
Technique

- Stand facing the ladder with the arms holding on at shoulder height.
- Have one foot on each cart equal distance from the centre line.
- Push both carts back extending the arms but keeping body upright with shoulders, hips and ankles all in alignment.
- Return to the starting position keeping an upright posture.

Tips

- Try to use your core strength to keep the pelvis stable.
- Keep the shoulders down.
- Imagine you are a statue being pushed back and forth on wheels.

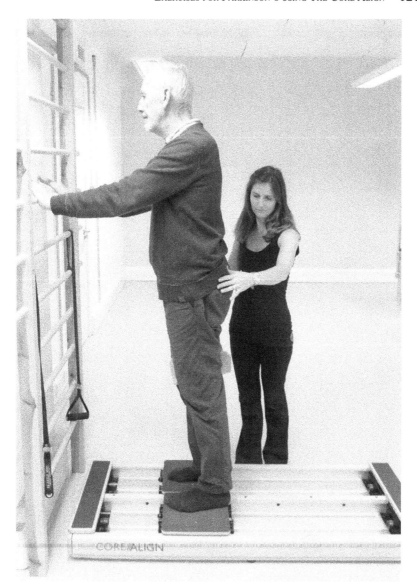

Figure 97

5 Curtsey
Technique

- Stand facing the ladder with the arms at waist height.
- Slide one cart back extending the arms and lifting the heel with slight flexion of the knee.

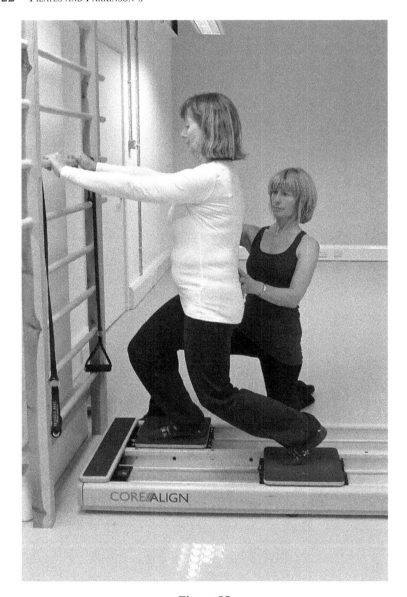

Figure 98

- Then drop down into a curtsey position with the knee positioned directly under the hip.
- Glide the cart back in whilst returning to the standing position.
- Alternate sides.

Tips

- Keep the pelvis stable throughout.

- Keep the knees aligned over the toes.
- Try not to round the shoulders as you move away from the ladder.
- Imagine you are dropping down to a curtsey with the posture of a ballet dancer: try to keep the spine completely straight and upper body relaxed.

6 Curtsey With Rotation
Technique

- Stand facing the ladder with your arms at waist height.
- Slide one cart back extending the arms and lifting the heel with slight flexion of the knee.
- Then take the opposite arm around to the side and rotating the upper body drop down into a curtsey position with your knee positioned directly under the hip.
- Glide the cart back in whilst returning to the standing position.
- Alternate sides.

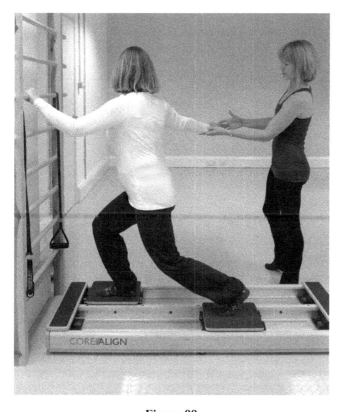

Figure 99

Tips

- Keep the pelvis stable throughout.
- Keep the knees aligned over the toes.
- Try to keep the extended arm just below shoulder height and follow the hand with your head.
- Try to achieve a relaxed flowing movement throughout this exercise, arms and legs should start and finish together.

7 Bird
Technique

- Stand facing away from the ladder.
- Hold the rope handles loosely with your arms by your sides.
- Slide forward on one cart bending the knee.
- Tilt your body forward whilst raising the arms out to the side keeping them slightly behind your torso.
- Engage your abdominal muscles as you return to the starting position.
- Repeat to the other side.

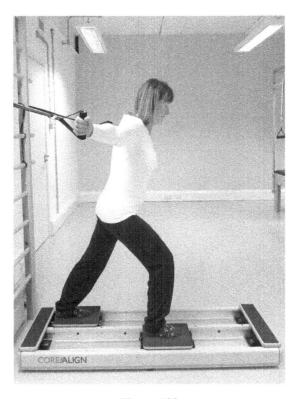

Figure 100

Tips

- Let the back heel lift slightly if needed.
- Keep the front knee over the toes.
- Keep the head in line with the spine.
- Use the abdominal muscles, not arms, on the return.
- Try to make a straight line from the shoulders to the back of your heels. Feel the stretch through the chest with the arms outstretched but relaxed – like a bird in flight.

Summary

- There are many different Pilates exercises out there, and certainly too many to include all of them in this book. If you know what you are supposed to be working on and why it will help, you and your instructor will be able to find the right exercises for you.
- Correct breathing and relaxation will improve lung function efficiency and help muscles to gently relax.
- Good shoulder and thoracic spine mobility will improve arm swing and trunk rotation during walking.
- Good stability around the scapulae, core and pelvis are required to allow smooth movement of the arms and legs.
- Exercises that involve stretching of the arms will help with reaching activities.
- Pilates exercises incorporate several different elements at once so mindfulness and dual tasking will improve.
- Exercises in prone, or lying on your tummy will stretch out tight muscle, encourage extension and inhibit flexion, which is really important for posture, BUT use them with caution, and if necessary, after advice.
- A good imagination and a good, well qualified instructor will allow you to translate matwork exercises into standing and walking which will ensure you have a wholly beneficial and meaningful exercise regime.
- Props can be an excellent addition to your workout, keeping it interesting and fun. Pilates machines in a fully equipped studio can also add another dimension to your workout.
- Don't move onto the next step until you have mastered the one you are on.
- Don't forget the feet, they can sometimes get stiff and tight with Parkinson's.

CHAPTER 10

Case Studies and Testimonials

Ray's Story

In February 2011 Ray, age 65 and retired, presented to his GP with a tremor of his right hand. He was diagnosed with early stage Parkinson's but no medication was indicated. Ray decided to come to us for a suitable Pilates regime to increase flexibility in stiff joints and muscles as well as maintaining his mobility and balance. He wanted to be as proactive as possible in managing this diagnosis and to stay in good physical condition being able to carry out his outdoor tasks with greater ease and less discomfort. Ray lives with his wife and they are both very active with two donkeys and a large garden and field to tend to.

What We Found

When we assessed Ray we found him to have a tremor of the right hand, tightness and weakness of the right shoulder with restricted movement, decreased hip mobility and weakness of the surrounding muscles, decreased core stability around the right side of his trunk, tightness of the right hamstrings, decreased ankle mobility, particularly on the right, poor trunk rotation and arm swing when walking and a stiff neck which he held in a poor position with his chin poking forwards. From these findings we can see that the muscles on the right side of his body were affected most by the Parkinson's. Ray also reported that occasional he "froze" when reaching an obstacle or doorway.

What We Worked On

We designed a Pilates exercise programme to improve joint mobility and muscle flexibility that also got Ray up into standing to work on his balance. Initially the programme was designed by the studio physiotherapist but was then taken over by another Pilates Instructor who was experienced in the management of Parkinson's. The instructor saw Ray in his own home so the programme was mainly matwork exercises. Initially Ray was reviewed every three months by the physiotherapist where an assessment was done of joints, muscles and balance so that any changes could be noted and the programme altered accordingly. With Ray we particularly worked on shoulder mobility using exercises such as *pelvic tilts with arms, the windmill, chicken wings* on the roller and the *dumb waiter*.

We wanted to increase thoracic spine mobility so he did exercises such as *cossack arms, bow and arrow and side lying arm* openings. To strengthen his hips we gave Ray the side lying leg exercises. We really noticed that initially when Ray did the *prone swimming* exercise, he couldn't lift his left arm up off the floor, as if it were stuck down with superglue! We felt this was because he lacked stability around his right abdominals and pelvis so we worked on all the pelvic stability exercises with movement of arms and legs incorporated. For example *single leg stretch*, which was also great to lengthen his hamstrings and *4 point swimming*. Ray's ankles were tight so we made sure he was stretching these at the end of his sessions as well has mobilising the joints of his feet manually during physiotherapy sessions. We also worked on Ray's neck giving him lots of gentle neck rotation and neck retractions using the small inflatable ball as well as back stabilisation exercises in sitting and prone. As the weeks and months went by Ray noticed that he became more flexible and strong.

At his physiotherapy assessment at 10 months he had full range of movement of his right shoulder, his ankles were much improved and he was able achieve child pose or back stretch comfortably, now able to get his bottom back on his heels whereas before he never could. When Ray did the *prone swimming* exercise he could now lift his left arm off the floor with ease and not as if it weighed a tonne. Ray was also pleased that the job of mending the sit on mower that in the past had taken hours and had left him with stiffness and pain for days now took only a couple of hours and he was left with no discomfort. He no longer experiences freezing during walking.

What Ray Does to Maintain His Ability

Ray continues to have weekly Pilates sessions and enjoys the challenge of more and more inventive exercises set by the instructor. With regular review (now only 6 monthly) from the physiotherapist we also keep a check on his balance and mobility, making sure he can step in all sorts of directions, patterns and speeds, dual tasking if necessary! At Ray's yearly appointment with the neurologist in June 2014, the consultant and Ray were very pleased that he had shown almost no deterioration since diagnosis in 2011.

Renato's Story

Renato, a 55-year-old Italian engineer living in the UK with his wife and three children was diagnosed with Parkinson's in 2006. His neurologists in Italy started him on Parkinson's medication and he also underwent deep brain stimulation in 2010. He came to our studio in March of 2014 for assessment by the physiotherapist with regards to appropriate exercises and a studio Pilates programme.

What We Found

His main complaint was that his left foot felt weak and stiff so as well as wishing to improve this he also wanted to stay as fit as possible. The physiotherapist assessed Renato and found very slight weakness throughout the muscle groups of the left leg, tightness of the left Achilles tendon and stiffness in the joints of the left foot. When she asked Renato to stand on one leg his toes would become very overactive and claw in an attempt to maintain balance. He was also found to have stiffness on neck flexion and rotation. Renato received 6 sessions of one to one physiotherapy combined with Pilates.

What We Worked On

The physiotherapist mobilised his foot using manual techniques and then we taught Renato a machine-based programme working on flexibility and strength, shoulder and back stability and trunk rotation. He particularly enjoyed *the mermaid stretch* on the reformer. The *footwork series* on the reformer was great, not only for mobilising and strengthening the feet but for the core as well. We got Renato standing and quickly went from exercises on 2 feet to performing shoulder and arm exercises on one foot or a balance board to increase the challenge. The foot exercises such as *doming*, picking objects up with his feet without the toes clawing and lifting the big toe up without the others and vice versa were very effective in getting the joints moving and waking up the small muscles of the feet. To improve neck movements we used the green ball exercises and strengthened the mid back with exercises lying on his front such as the diamond press and dart.

What We Noticed

After 6 sessions with the physiotherapist Renato joined the normal studio sessions under the supervision of experienced instructors as it was felt he was ready to progress to a different programme, requiring less hands on from a physiotherapist. In July 2014 he was reviewed by the physiotherapist who found that his left Achilles tendon was no longer tight and he had no stiffness of the joints of the left foot a tall.

What Renato Does to Maintain His Ability

Renato continues to attend the studio each week and is reviewed by the physiotherapist every 6–8 weeks to monitor the foot and balance activities and also to progress the Pilates exercise programme to make it more challenging.

Rita's Story

Rita first noticed symptoms in the spring of 2012, initially it was subtle things such as a small tremor affecting her manual dexterity when undoing buttons, sewing or pricking out seedlings. She found that simple things took a long time and more concentration. She had always led a very active life then suddenly even walking became difficult and she became tired very easily. She had recognised some of the symptoms as her mother had suffered with Parkinson's, so although her GP had assured her that this disease was not usually associated with a genetic tie she arranged for her to see a neurologist. She was diagnosed with Parkinson's in December 2012.

What We Found

Rita first came to the Pilates studio in January 2013. Although she was a fairly agile person naturally, she had developed a shuffling gait, tightness down the whole of her left side, restricted trunk rotation to the left and slightly rounded shoulders. Her neck extensors were tight and caused her to hold her head in a very tense position. The arches of her feet were also very tight and caused discomfort and cramping.

What We Worked On

We started work on her core strength initially and added some exercises to help with co-ordination such as *windmills* and the *bugs* exercise on roller as well as some neck relaxing exercises with a soft green ball (slightly deflated). These exercises made a huge difference to how Rita felt and so she bought a soft ball and roller to use at home.

We then added some exercises to open her chest and improve the strength of her back extensors. To try and improve her gait and reduce the shuffling we attached long springs to the Trapeze table and did some bow and arrow movements as well as some simple swinging of the arms whilst turning her head which she practiced at home. We also used the Reformer for leg work both supine (lying on her back) for hip and knee joint mobility, and side lying for hip extensor work to help with the follow through of her gait.

What Rita does to maintain her ability

As Rita's core strength improved she was able to move onto more interesting exercises and now makes particularly good use of the Core Align. The standing gait exercises with rotation are particularly beneficial as is the *kneeling back stretch with rotation*.

Rita attends the studio twice weekly, we challenge her with new exercises and she manages to execute and pick them up skillfully.

What We Noticed

Although Rita still has to work hard to maintain rotation on her left side she has greatly improved her coordination, has wonderful flexibility in her hamstrings and her balance and overall mobility has improved enormously. Rita found the back stability exerices difficult to start with but persevered and feels she has now lost the "round shouldered look".

Testimonials

I have attended Pilates (with physiotherapy) for several months. The Pilates expertise combined with physiotherapy has enabled the programme to be tailored to my needs. Pilates has markedly benefited me in terms of flexibility and balance and I feel I have significantly improved bodily strength and posture. No two sessions have been the same, building each time on my improving capabilities. The exercises are taught in a friendly, effective and confidence inducing manner. All the studio team are impressive and highly professional teachers. Thank you for everything you have done: you really have made such a difference and, although far from happy with the diagnosis, I feel I am doing something to help myself. You have encouraged me every step of the way and I am so grateful. *Ray*

I started Pilates sessions in January 2013 and discovered that my coordination was very poor, I remember being asked to swing my arms and march like a soldier and was shocked to discover that I couldn't do this simple movement. I practiced marching around the house, and still do if I feel my body is stiffening and needs reminding.

I found that all the exercises helped with awareness of my body's movement and noticed that my left side was always weaker than the right. My mobility has improved enormously and I now am able to enjoy walks of 3 or 4 miles for pleasure.

I recently had abdominal surgery and missed my classes for several weeks; I was surprised at how quickly I lost mobility and strength and how important it is for me to practice the exercises at least twice a week. Sometimes I suffer pain/stiffness in my sides and back so I lie on the floor and do some Pilates exercises and relaxation for a few minutes and this leaves me pain free with no need to take analgesics.

My Pilates instructor has helped me in so many ways for example my walking, core strength, balance, concentration, relaxation and body awareness. And of course humour when I find a way to 'cheat' an exercise! *Rita*

Pilates isn't going to cure me of Parkinson's but it has made a big difference to how I feel, how I stand and walk and what I can do. Six years on from my initial diagnosis I go sailing, play table tennis and take regular walks.

Karen Pearce and her assistants at the Pilates Studio developed a programme of exercises to stretch and relax my back, which without regular sessions would stiffen up and occasionally go into spasm.

Of course, the drugs I take play a crucial part in keeping me on the move but I am convinced that without Pilates they would be a lot less effective. *Graham*

I have found Pilates to be an excellent form of exercise, and continue to find it therapeutic 16 years after being diagnosed at the age of 54. I go to classes locally, twice a week in winter and once a week in summer. Pilates suits me personally more than yoga and other indoor gym exercises. I was very fit when I was diagnosed, and have tried to remain so. Three years ago I cycled 1600 miles in 28 days to raise money for Pedal for Parkinson's. I seem to respond well to medication, I play the violin (badly) but find it interesting that I can still play. *Mark*

Resources

Parkinson's UK
215 Vauxhall Bridge Road, London SW1V 1EJ
0808 800 0303
www.parkinsons.org.uk

Association of Physiotherapists in Parkinson's Disease Europe
www.appde.eu

Chartered Society of Physiotherapists
14 Bedford Row London, WC1R 4ED.
020 7306 6666
www.csp.org.uk

The Physiotherapy and Pilates Rehabilitation Centre
Unit 2, Neads Court, Knowles Road, Clevedon, North Somerset. BS21 7XS
www.sarahsessaphysio.co.uk
www.thepilatesstudio.co.uk

The Pilates Studio, Taunton
33 – 39 Bridge Street, Taunton TA1 1TP
01823 423146
www.thepilatesstudio.co.uk

Illustrations
www.eileen-hall.com

About the Authors

Sarah Sessa BSc (Hons) Physiotherapy

Sarah qualified as a physiotherapist from University College London (UCL) in 1995. She went on to work at The Middlesex and UCL hospitals until 2002 where she gained invaluable experience working in trauma and ortho-paedics, elderly care, amputees, neurology, oncology, HIV, general medical wards, accident and emergency and intensive care. During that period she also spent time at the National Hospital for Neurological Diseases, Queen Square working on the Acute Brain Injury Unit. She developed a keen interest in rehabilitation within the areas of neurology, oncology and complex reha-bilitation. After 2002 Sarah worked as a senior rehabilitation physiotherapist on the stroke unit and oncology wards at the Oxford Radcliffe Hospitals and after leaving Oxford for Somerset she went on to work St Margaret's Hos-pice in Taunton providing rehabilitation within palliative care.

Sarah started doing Pilates herself in the late 1990's and increasingly saw the benefits it could have within the area of rehabilitation so decided to do a teacher training course. She qualified as a Pilates Instructor in affil-iation with Alan Herdman at the Pilates Studio in Taunton in 2009. She set up her own business, Sarah Sessa Physiotherapy from home and saw a variety of clients: from musicians to horse riders who wanted a person-alised Pilates programme and those with neurological conditions such as Parkinson's, stroke, multiple sclerosis and motor neurone disease who ben-efited enormously from a Pilates programme combined with physiother-apy. She now runs the Physiotherapy and Pilates Rehabilitation Centre in Clevedon with Karen working closely with the Pilates instructors to pro-vide bespoke rehabilitation and Pilates programmes and also offers phys-iotherapy for neurological and other medical conditions.

Sarah also lectures on the Centre's teacher training programme and is currently studying for her MSc at the University of the West of England.

Karen Pearce

After training at The Royal Ballet School Karen went on to have a career as a professional ballet dancer, dancing soloist and principle roles with

Kiel Ballet Company, Germany and Northern Ballet Theatre in England. In the late 1990's, after moving to Somerset and having three children, she trained and qualified as a Pilates Instructor with Alan Herdman in London. Karen set up a small Pilates studio in her house in Somerset in 1999 then, due to demand, quickly realised that she needed to expand. She is now the Founder and Director of The Pilates Studios (SW) Limited, runs studios in Taunton, Bristol and Clevedon and runs a Pilates Teacher Training Course in affiliation with Alan Herdman.

Karen had always been aware of the benefits of Pilates as a dancer although it had been used mainly as a source of rehabilitation following injury for herself and fellow dancers. It wasn't until she started to teach Pilates that she realised how beneficial it could be for all, whether fit, young, old or as a method of rehabilitation.

In her 16 years of teaching Pilates Karen has built a reputation with local physiotherapists, osteopaths and surgeons who regularly refer patients to her studios, together with teaching dancers, athletes and professional sports people such as members of Somerset County Cricket Club.

Acknowledgements

We would like to thank our families for all their support and encouragement throughout this process.

Thank you to the brilliant physiotherapist Bhanu Ramaswamy, FCSP for her invaluable advice and feedback.

Thank you to Alan Herdman for being a truly inspirational mentor.

Thank you to Eileen Hall for the stunning drawings.

Thanks to our models Rita McClure and Ray Spurgeon who attend Pilates regularly and are wonderful examples of people living with Parkinson's.

Thank you to Kate Lewis, our matwork model who has given so much of her time to help us with this book.

Thank you to Ben, Jo Pritchard (MCSP), Mark, Ray and Bhanu Ramaswamy for proof reading, commenting and pointing out things we might have missed!

Finally we would like to offer special thanks to our clients with Parkinson's who have worked so hard in our studios and inspired us to write this book.

Notes

1. Pilates J and Miller J 1945 Pilates' Return to Life Through Contrology
2. Aragon et al. 2007 The Professional's Guide to Parkinson's Disease. 3, 106–107, 109, 118 (2007)
3. Parkinson's UK. 2013 What is Parkinson's. http://www.parkinsons.org.uk/content/what-parkinsons
4. Speelman A et al. 2011. How Might Physical Activity Benefit Patients with Parkinson's Disease. Nature Reviews Neurology 7, 528–534
5. Keus SHJ, Munneke M, Graziano M, et al. European Physiotherapy Guidelines for Parkinson's disease. 2014: KNGF/ParkinsonNet, the Netherlands
6. Withers G and E et al. 2009 Modified Pilates Rehabilitation Programme (manual): Pilates and Neurology.
7. Parkinson's UK 2013. http://www.parkinsons.org.uk/content/complementary-therapies-and-parkinsons-booklet.
8. Hudson K. 2013 Pilates Predictions: Health Club Management. 56–58. www.healthclubmanagement.co.uk/digital)
9. Royer et al. 2007 Pilates for People with Parkinson's Disease. Balanced Body Pilates COREterly. (Summer)
10. Hodges et al, 1999. Is There a Role for Transversus Abdominus in Lumbo-Pelvic Stability? Manual Therapy 4(2) 74–86.
11. Morris M et al. 2010. Striding out With Parkinson Disease: Evidence-Based Physical Therapy for Gait Disorders. Physical Therapy 90, 280–288

Printed in the USA
CPSIA information can be obtained
at www.ICGtesting.com
JSHW051458221024
72172JS00011B/101

9 781913 274122